THE EVOLUTION OF MODERN MEDICINE A SERIES OF LECTURES DELIVERED AT YALE UNIVERSITY ON THE SILLIMAN FOUNDATION IN APRIL, 1913 • OSLER, WILLIAM

THE SILLIMAN FOUNDATION 1
PREFACE 2

CHAPTER I — ORIGIN OF MEDICINE 3
INTRODUCTION 3
ORIGIN OF MEDICINE 5
EGYPTIAN MEDICINE 6
ASSYRIAN AND BABYLONIAN MEDICINE 8
HEBREW MEDICINE 12
CHINESE AND JAPANESE MEDICINE 13

CHAPTER II — GREEK MEDICINE 14
ASKLEPIOS 17
HIPPOCRATES AND THE HIPPOCRATIC WRITINGS 20
ALEXANDRIAN SCHOOL 25
GALEN 26

CHAPTER III — MEDIAEVAL MEDICINE 28
SOUTH ITALIAN SCHOOL 29
BYZANTINE MEDICINE 30
ARABIAN MEDICINE 30
THE RISE OF THE UNIVERSITIES 34
MEDIAEVAL MEDICAL STUDIES 37
MEDIAEVAL PRACTICE 38
ASTROLOGY AND DIVINATION 38

CHAPTER IV — THE RENAISSANCE AND THE RISE OF ANATOMY AND PHYSIOLOGY 40
PARACELSUS 42
VESALIUS 46
HARVEY 50

CHAPTER V — THE RISE AND DEVELOPMENT OF MODERN MEDICINE 54
INTERNAL SECRETIONS 61
CHEMISTRY 61

CHAPTER VI — THE RISE OF PREVENTIVE MEDICINE 62
SANITATION 63
TUBERCULOSIS 68

Publisher's Note

Purchase of this book entitles you to a free trial membership in the publisher's book club at www.rarebooksclub.com. (Time limited offer.) Simply enter the barcode number from the back cover onto the membership form on our home page. The book club entitles you to select from millions of books at no additional charge. You can also download a digital copy of this and related books to read on the go. Simply enter the title or subject onto the search form to find them.

Note: This is an historic book. Pages numbers, where present in the text, refer to the first edition of the book and may also be in indexes.

If you have any questions, could you please be so kind as to consult our Frequently Asked Questions page at www.rarebooksclub.com/faqs.cfm? You are also welcome to contact us there.
Publisher: General Books LLC™, Memphis, TN, USA, 2012. ISBN: 9781770457591.
Proofreading: pgdp.net

❦ ❦ ❦ ❦ ❦ ❦ ❦ ❦

THE EVOLUTION OF MODERN MEDICINE

A SERIES OF LECTURES DELIVERED AT YALE UNIVERSITY

ON THE SILLIMAN FOUNDATION

IN APRIL, 1913

by William Osler

THE SILLIMAN FOUNDATION

IN the year 1883 a legacy of eighty thousand dollars was left to the President and Fellows of Yale College in the city of New Haven, to be held in trust, as a gift from her children, in memory of their beloved and honored mother, Mrs. Hepsa Ely Silliman.

On this foundation Yale College was requested and directed to establish an annual course of lectures designed to illustrate the presence and providence, the wisdom and goodness of God, as manifested in the natural and moral world. These were to be designated as the Mrs. Hepsa Ely Silliman Memorial Lectures. It was the belief of the testator that any orderly presentation of the facts of nature or history contributed to the end of this foundation more effectively than any attempt to emphasize the elements of doctrine or of creed; and he therefore provided that lectures on dogmatic or polemical theology should be excluded from the scope of this foundation, and that the subjects should be selected rather from the domains of natural science and history, giving special prominence to astronomy, chemistry, geology and anatomy.

It was further directed that each annual course should be made the basis of a volume to form part of a series constituting a memorial to Mrs. Silliman. The memorial fund came into the possession of the Corporation of Yale University in the year 1901; and the present volume constitutes the tenth of the series of memorial lectures.

PREFACE

THE manuscript of Sir William Osler's lectures on the "Evolution of Modern Medicine," delivered at Yale University in April, 1913, on the Silliman Foundation, was immediately turned in to the Yale University Press for publication. Duly set in type, proofs in galley form had been submitted to him and despite countless interruptions he had already corrected and revised a number of the galleys when the great war came. But with the war on, he threw himself with energy and devotion into the military and public duties which devolved upon him and so never completed his proofreading and intended alterations. The careful corrections which Sir William made in the earlier galleys show that the lectures were dictated, in the first instance, as loose memoranda for oral delivery rather than as finished compositions for the eye, while maintaining throughout the logical continuity and the engaging con moto which were so characteristic of his literary style. In revising the lectures for publication, therefore, the editors have merely endeavored to carry out, with care and befitting reverence, the indications supplied in the earlier galleys by Sir William himself. In supplying dates and references which were lacking, his preferences as to editions and readings have been borne in mind. The slight alterations made, the adaptation of the text to the eye, detract nothing from the original freshness of the work.

In a letter to one of the editors, Osler described these lectures as "an aeroplane flight over the progress of medicine through the ages." They are, in effect, a sweeping panoramic survey of the whole vast field, covering wide areas at a rapid pace, yet with an extraordinary variety of detail. The slow, painful character of the evolution of medicine from the fearsome, superstitious mental complex of primitive man, with his amulets, healing gods and disease demons, to the ideal of a clear-eyed rationalism is traced with faith and a serene sense of continuity. The author saw clearly and felt deeply that the men who have made an idea or discovery viable and valuable to humanity are the deserving men; he has made the great names shine out, without any depreciation of the important work of lesser men and without cluttering up his narrative with the tedious prehistory of great discoveries or with shrill claims to priority. Of his skill in differentiating the sundry "strains" of medicine, there is specific witness in each section. Osler's wide culture and control of the best available literature of his subject permitted him to range the ampler aether of Greek medicine or the earth-fettered schools of today with equal mastery; there is no quickset of pedantry between the author and the reader. The illustrations (which he had doubtless planned as fully for the last as for the earlier chapters) are as he left them; save that, lacking legends, these have been supplied and a few which could not be identified have with regret been omitted. The original galley proofs have been revised and corrected from different viewpoints by Fielding H. Garrison, Harvey Cushing, Edward C. Streeter and latterly by Leonard L. Mackall (Savannah, Ga.), whose zeal and persistence in the painstaking verification of citations and references cannot be too highly commended.

In the present revision, a number of important corrections, most of them based upon the original MS., have been made by Dr. W.W. Francis (Oxford), Dr. Charles Singer (London), Dr. E.C. Streeter, Mr. L.L. Mackall and others.

This work, composed originally for a lay audience and for popular consumption, will be to the aspiring medical student and the hardworking practitioner a lift into the blue, an inspiring vista or "Pisgah-sight" of the evolution of medicine, a realization of what devotion, perseverance, valor and ability on the part of physicians have contributed to this progress, and of the creditable part which our profession has played in the general development of science.

The editors have no hesitation in presenting these lectures to the profession and to the reading public as one of the most characteristic productions of the best-balanced, best-equipped, most sagacious and most lovable of all modern physicians.

F.H.G.

BUT on that account, I say, we ought not to reject the ancient Art, as if it were not, and had not been properly founded, because it did not attain accuracy in all things, but rather, since it is capable of reaching to the greatest exactitude by reasoning, to receive it and admire its discoveries, made from a state of great ignorance, and as having been well and properly made, and not from chance. (Hippocrates, On Ancient Medicine, Adams edition, Vol. 1, 1849, p. 168.)

THE true and lawful goal of the sciences is none other than this: that human life be endowed with new discoveries and powers. (Francis Bacon, Novum Organum, Aphorisms, LXXXI, Spedding's translation.)

A GOLDEN thread has run throughout the history of the world, consecutive and continuous, the work of the best men in successive ages. From point to point it still runs, and when near you feel it as the clear and bright and searchingly irresistible light which Truth throws forth when great minds conceive it. (Walter Moxon, Pilocereus Senilis and Other Papers, 1887, p. 4.)

FOR the mind depends so much on the temperament and disposition of the bodily organs that, if it is possible to find a means of rendering men wiser and cleverer than they have hitherto been, I believe that it is in medicine that it must be sought. It is true that the medicine which is now in vogue contains little of which the utility is remarkable; but, without having any intention of decrying it, I am sure that there is no one, even among those who make its study a profession, who does not confess that all that men know is almost nothing in comparison with what remains to be known; and that we could be free of an infinitude of maladies both of body and mind, and even also possibly of the infirmities of age, if we had sufficient knowledge of their causes, and of all the remedies with which nature has provided us. (Descartes: Discourse on the Method, Philosophical Works. Translated by E. S. Haldane and G. R. T. Ross. Vol. I, Cam. Univ. Press, 1911, p. 120.)

CHAPTER I — ORIGIN OF MEDICINE

INTRODUCTION

SAIL to the Pacific with some Ancient Mariner, and traverse day by day that silent sea until you reach a region never before furrowed by keel where a tiny island, a mere speck on the vast ocean, has just risen from the depths, a little coral reef capped with green, an atoll, a mimic earth, fringed with life, built up through countless ages by life on the remains of life that has passed away. And now, with wings of fancy, join Ianthe in the magic car of Shelley, pass the eternal gates of the flaming ramparts of the world and see his vision:

Below lay stretched the boundless Universe!
There, far as the remotest line
That limits swift imagination's flight,
Unending orbs mingled in mazy motion,
Immutably fulfilling
Eternal Nature's law.
Above, below, around,
The circling systems formed
A wilderness of harmony.
(Daemon of the World, Pt. I.)

And somewhere, 'as fast and far the chariot flew," amid the mighty globes would be seen a tiny speck, "earth's distant orb," one of "the smallest lights that twinkle in the heavens." Alighting, Ianthe would find something she had probably not seen elsewhere in her magic flight—life, everywhere encircling the sphere. And as the little coral reef out of a vast depth had been built up by generations of polyzoa, so she would see that on the earth, through illimitable ages, successive generations of animals and plants had left in stone their imperishable records: and at the top of the series she would meet the thinking, breathing creature known as man. Infinitely little as is the architect of the atoll in proportion to the earth on which it rests, the polyzoon, I doubt not, is much larger relatively than is man in proportion to the vast systems of the Universe, in which he represents an ultra-microscopic atom less ten thousand times than the tiniest of the "gay motes that people the sunbeams." Yet, with colossal audacity, this thinking atom regards himself as the anthropocentric pivot around which revolve the eternal purposes of the Universe. Knowing not whence he came, why he is here, or whither he is going, man feels himself of supreme importance, and certainly is of interest—to himself. Let us hope that he has indeed a potency and importance out of all proportion to his somatic insignificance. We know of toxins of such strength that an amount too infinitesimal to be gauged may kill; and we know that 'the unit adopted in certain scientific work is the amount of emanation produced by one million-millionth of a grain of radium, a quantity which itself has a volume of less than a million-millionth of a cubic millimetre and weighs a million million times less than an exceptionally delicate chemical balance will turn to" (Soddy, 1912). May not man be the radium of the Universe? At any rate let us not worry about his size. For us he is a very potent creature, full of interest, whose mundane story we are only beginning to unravel.

Civilization is but a filmy fringe on the history of man. Go back as far as his records carry us and the story written on stone is of yesterday in comparison with the vast epochs of time which modern studies demand for his life on the earth. For two millions (some hold even three millions) of years man lived and moved and had his being in a world very different from that upon which we look out. There appear, indeed, to have been various types of man, some as different from us as we are from the anthropoid apes. What upstarts of yesterday are the Pharaohs in comparison with the men who survived the tragedy of the glacial period! The ancient history of man—only now beginning to be studied—dates from the Pliocene or Miocene period; the modern history, as we know it, embraces that brief space of time that has elapsed since the earliest Egyptian and Babylonian records were made. This has to be borne in mind in connection with the present mental status of man, particularly in his outlook upon nature. In his thoughts and in his attributes, mankind at large is controlled by inherited beliefs and impulses, which countless thousands of years have ingrained like instinct. Over vast regions of the earth today, magic, amulets, charms, incantations are the chief weapons of defense against a malignant nature; and in disease, the practice of Asa(*) is comparatively novel and unusual; in days of illness many millions more still seek their gods rather than the physicians. In an upward path man has had to work out for himself a relationship with his fellows and with nature. He sought in the supernatural an explanation of the pressing phenomena of life, peopling the world with spiritual beings, deifying objects of nature, and assigning to them benign or malign influences, which might be invoked or propitiated. Primitive priest, physician and philosopher were one, and struggled, on the one hand, for the recognition of certain practices forced on him by experience, and on the other, for the recognition of mystical agencies which control the dark, "uncharted region" about him—to use Prof. Gilbert Murray's phrase—and were responsible for everything he could not understand, and particularly for the mysteries of disease. Pliny remarks that physic "was early fathered upon the gods"; and to the ordinary non-medical mind, there is still something mysterious about sickness, something outside the ordinary standard.

(*) II Chronicles xvi, 12.

Modern anthropologists claim that both religion and medicine took origin in magic, "that spiritual protoplasm," as

Miss Jane Harrison calls it. To primitive man, magic was the setting in motion of a spiritual power to help or to hurt the individual, and early forms may still be studied in the native races. This power, or "mana," as it is called, while possessed in a certain degree by all, may be increased by practice. Certain individuals come to possess it very strongly: among native Australians today it is still deliberately cultivated. Magic in healing seeks to control the demons, or forces; causing disease; and in a way it may be thus regarded as a "lineal ancestor of modern science" (Whetham), which, too, seeks to control certain forces, no longer, however, regarded as supernatural.

Primitive man recognized many of these superhuman agencies relating to disease, such as the spirits of the dead, either human or animal, independent disease demons, or individuals who might act by controlling the spirits or agencies of disease. We see this today among the negroes of the Southern States. A Hoodoo put upon a negro may, if he knows of it, work upon him so powerfully through the imagination that he becomes very ill indeed, and only through a more powerful magic exercised by someone else can the Hoodoo be taken off.

To primitive man life seemed "full of sacred presences" (Walter Pater) connected with objects in nature, or with incidents and epochs in life, which he began early to deify, so that, until a quite recent period, his story is largely associated with a pantheon of greater and lesser gods, which he has manufactured wholesale. Xenophanes was the earliest philosopher to recognize man's practice of making gods in his own image and endowing them with human faculties and attributes; the Thracians, he said, made their gods blue-eyed and red-haired, the Ethiopians, snub-nosed and black, while, if oxen and lions and horses had hands and could draw, they would represent their gods as oxen and lions and horses. In relation to nature and to disease, all through early history we find a pantheon full to repletion, bearing testimony no less to the fertility of man's imagination than to the hopes and fears which led him, in his exodus from barbarism, to regard his gods as "pillars of fire by night, and pillars of cloud by day."

Even so late a religion as that of Numa was full of little gods to be invoked on special occasions—Vatican, who causes the infant to utter his first cry, Fabulinus, who prompts his first word, Cuba, who keeps him quiet in his cot, Domiduca, who watches over one's safe home-coming (Walter Pater); and Numa believed that all diseases came from the gods and were to be averted by prayer and sacrifice. Besides the major gods, representatives of Apollo, AEsculapius and Minerva, there were scores of lesser ones who could be invoked for special diseases. It is said that the young Roman mother might appeal to no less than fourteen goddesses, from Juno Lucina to Prosa and Portvorta (Withington). Temples were erected to the Goddess of Fever, and she was much invoked. There is extant a touching tablet erected by a mourning mother and inscribed:

Febri divae, Febri
Sancte, Febri magnae
Camillo amato pro
Filio meld effecto. Posuit.

It is marvellous what a long line of superhuman powers, major and minor, man has invoked against sickness. In Swinburne's words:

God by God flits past in thunder till his glories turn to shades,
God by God bears wondering witness how his Gospel flames and
    fades;
More was each of these, while yet they were, than man their
    servant seemed;
Dead are all of these, and man survives who made them while he
    dreamed.

Most of them have been benign and helpful gods. Into the dark
    chapters relating to demonical possession and to witchcraft we
    cannot here enter. They make one cry out with Lucretius (Bk. V):

O genus infelix humanum, talia divis
Cum tribuit facta atque iras adjunxit acerbas!
Quantos tum gemitus ipsi sibi, quantaque nobis
Vulnera, quas lacrimas peperere minoribu' nostris.

In every age, and in every religion there has been justification for his bitter words, "tantum religio potuit suadere malorum"—"Such wrongs Religion in her train doth bring"—yet, one outcome of "a belief in spiritual beings"—as Tylor defines religion—has been that man has built an altar of righteousness in his heart. The comparative method applied to the study of his religious growth has shown how man's thoughts have widened in the unceasing purpose which runs through his spiritual no less than his physical evolution. Out of the spiritual protoplasm of magic have evolved philosopher and physician, as well as priest. Magic and religion control the uncharted sphere—the supernatural, the superhuman: science seeks to know the world, and through knowing, to control it. Ray Lankester remarks that Man is Nature's rebel, and goes on to say: "The mental qualities which have developed in Man, though traceable in a vague and rudimentary condition in some of his animal associates, are of such an unprecedented power and so far dominate everything else in his activities as a living organism, that they have to a very large extent, if not entirely, cut him off from the general operation of that process of Natural Selection and survival of the fittest which up to their appearance had been the law of the living world. They justify the view that Man forms a new departure in the gradual unfolding of Nature's predestined scheme. Knowledge, reason, self-consciousness, will, are the attributes of Man."[1] It has been a slow and gradual growth, and not until within the past century has science organized knowledge—so searched out the secrets of Nature, as to control her powers, limit her scope and transform her energies. The victory is so recent that the mental attitude of the race is not yet adapted to the change. A large proportion of our fellow creatures still regard nature as a playground for demons and spirits to be exorcised or invoked.

(1) Sir E. Ray Lankester: Romanes Lecture, "Nature and Man,"
Oxford Univ. Press, 1905, p. 21.

Side by side, as substance and shadow—"in the dark backward and abysm of time," in the dawn of the great civilizations of Egypt and Babylon, in the bright morning of Greece, and in the full noontide of modern life, together have grown up these two diametrically opposite views of man's relation to nature, and more particularly of his personal relation to the agencies of disease.

The purpose of this course of lectures is to sketch the main features of the growth of these two dominant ideas, to show how they have influenced man at the different periods of his evolution, how the lamp of reason, so early lighted in his soul, burning now bright, now dim, has never, even in his darkest period, been wholly extinguished, but retrimmed and refurnished by his indomitable energies, now shines more and more towards the perfect day. It is a glorious chapter in history, in which those who have eyes to see may read the fulfilment of the promise of Eden, that one day man should not only possess the earth, but that he should have dominion over it! I propose to take an aeroplane flight through the centuries, touching only on the tall peaks from which may be had a panoramic view of the epochs through which we pass.

ORIGIN OF MEDICINE

MEDICINE arose out of the primal sympathy of man with man; out of the desire to help those in sorrow, need and sickness.

In the primal sympathy
Which having been must ever be;
In the soothing thoughts that spring

Out of human suffering.

The instinct of self-preservation, the longing to relieve a loved one, and above all, the maternal passion—for such it is—gradually softened the hard race of man—tum genus humanum primum mollescere coepit. In his marvellous sketch of the evolution of man, nothing illustrates more forcibly the prescience of Lucretius than the picture of the growth of sympathy: "When with cries and gestures they taught with broken words that 'tis right for all men to have pity on the weak." I heard the well-known medical historian, the late Dr. Payne, remark that "the basis of medicine is sympathy and the desire to help others, and whatever is done with this end must be called medicine."

The first lessons came to primitive man by injuries, accidents, bites of beasts and serpents, perhaps for long ages not appreciated by his childlike mind, but, little by little, such experiences crystallized into useful knowledge. The experiments of nature made clear to him the relation of cause and effect, but it is not likely, as Pliny suggests, that he picked up his earliest knowledge from the observation of certain practices in animals, as the natural phlebotomy of the plethoric hippopotamus, or the use of emetics from the dog, or the use of enemata from the ibis. On the other hand, Celsus is probably right in his account of the origin of rational medicine. "Some of the sick on account of their eagerness took food on the first day, some on account of loathing abstained; and the disease in those who refrained was more relieved. Some ate during a fever, some a little before it, others after it had subsided, and those who had waited to the end did best. For the same reason some at the beginning of an illness used a full diet, others a spare, and the former were made worse. Occurring daily, such things impressed careful men, who noted what had best helped the sick, then began to prescribe them. In this way medicine had its rise from the experience of the recovery of some, of the death of others, distinguishing the hurtful from the salutary

things" (Book I). The association of ideas was suggestive—the plant eyebright was used for centuries in diseases of the eye because a black speck in the flower suggested the pupil of the eye. The old herbals are full of similar illustrations upon which, indeed, the so-called doctrine of signatures depends. Observation came, and with it an ever widening experience. No society so primitive without some evidence of the existence of a healing art, which grew with its growth, and became part of the fabric of its organization.

With primitive medicine, as such, I cannot deal, but I must refer to the oldest existing evidence of a very extraordinary practice, that of trephining. Neolithic skulls with disks of bone removed have been found in nearly all parts of the world. Many careful studies have been made of this procedure, particularly by the great anatomist and surgeon, Paul Broca, and M. Lucas-Championniere has covered the subject in a monograph.(2) Broca suggests that the trephining was done by scratching or scraping, but, as Lucas-Championniere holds, it was also done by a series of perforations made in a circle with flint instruments, and a round piece of skull in this way removed; traces of these drill-holes have been found. The operation was done for epilepsy, infantile convulsions, headache, and various cerebral diseases believed to be caused by confined demons, to whom the hole gave a ready method of escape.

(2) Lucas-Championniere:
Trepanation neolithique, Paris, 1912.

The practice is still extant. Lucas-Championniere saw a Kabyle thoubib who told him that it was quite common among his tribe; he was the son of a family of trephiners, and had undergone the operation four times, his father twelve times; he had three brothers also experts; he did not consider it a dangerous operation. He did it most frequently for pain in the head, and occasionally for fracture.

The operation was sometimes performed upon animals. Shepherds trephined sheep for the staggers. We may say that the modern decompression operation, so much in vogue, is the oldest known surgical procedure.

EGYPTIAN MEDICINE

OUT of the ocean of oblivion, man emerges in history in a highly civilized state on the banks of the Nile, some sixty centuries ago. After millenniums of a gradual upward progress, which can be traced in the records of the stone age, civilization springs forth Minerva-like, complete, and highly developed, in the Nile Valley. In this sheltered, fertile spot, neolithic man first raised himself above his kindred races of the Mediterranean basin, and it is suggested that by the accidental discovery of copper Egypt "forged the instruments that raised civilization out of the slough of the Stone Age" (Elliot Smith). Of special interest to us is the fact that one of the best-known names of this earliest period is that of a physician—guide, philosopher and friend of the king—a man in a position of wide trust and importance. On leaving Cairo, to go up the Nile, one sees on the right in the desert behind Memphis a terraced pyramid 190 feet in height, "the first large structure of stone known in history." It is the royal tomb of Zoser, the first of a long series with which the Egyptian monarchy sought "to adorn the coming bulk of death." The design of this is attributed to Imhotep, the first figure of a physician to stand out clearly from the mists of antiquity. "In priestly wisdom, in magic, in the formulation of wise proverbs, in medicine and architecture, this remarkable figure of Zoser's reign left so notable a reputation that his name was never forgotten, and 2500 years after his death he had become a God of Medicine, in whom the Greeks, who called him Imouthes, recognized their own AEsculapius."(3) He became a popular god, not only healing men when alive, but taking good care of them in the journeys after death. The facts about this medicinae primus inventor, as he has been called, may be gathered from Kurt Sethe's study.(4) He seems to have corresponded very much to the Greek Asklepios. As a god he is met with comparatively late, between 700 and 332 B.C. Numerous bronze figures of him remain. The oldest memorial mentioning him is a statue of one of his priests, Amasis (No. 14765 in the British Museum). Ptolemy V dedicated to him a temple on the island of Philae. His cult increased much in later days, and a special temple was dedicated to him near Memphis Sethe suggests that the cult of Imhotep gave the inspiration to the Hermetic literature. The association of Imhotep with the famous temple at Edfu is of special interest.

(3) Breasted: A History of the Ancient Egyptians, Scribner,
New York, 1908, p. 104.

(4) K. Sethe: Imhotep, der Asklepios der Aegypter, Leipzig,
1909 (Untersuchungen, etc., ed. Sethe, Vol. II, No. 4).

Egypt became a centre from which civilization spread to the other peoples of the Mediterranean. For long centuries, to be learned in all the wisdom of the Egyptians meant the possession of all knowledge. We must come to the land of the Nile for the origin of many of man's most distinctive and highly cherished beliefs. Not only is there a magnificent material civilization, but in records so marvellously preserved in stone we may see, as in a glass, here clearly, there darkly, the picture of man's search after righteousness, the earliest impressions of his moral awakening, the beginnings of the strife in which he has always been engaged for social justice and for the recognition of the rights of the individual. But above all, earlier and more strongly than in any other people, was developed the faith that looked through death, to which, to this day, the noblest of their monuments bear an enduring testimony. With all this, it is not surprising to find a growth in the knowledge of practical medicine; but Egyptian civilization illustrates how crude and primitive may remain a knowledge of disease when conditioned by erroneous views of its nature. At first, the priest and physician were identified, and medicine never became fully dissociated from religion. Only in the later periods did a special group of physicians arise who were not members of priestly colleges.(6) Maspero states that the Egyptians believed that disease and death were not natural and inevitable, but caused by some malign influence which could use any agency, natural or invisible, and very often belonged to the invisible world. "Often, though, it belongs to the invisible world, and only reveals itself by the malignity of its attacks: it is a god, a spirit, the soul of a dead man, that has cunningly entered a living person, or that throws itself upon him with irresistible violence. Once in possession of the body, the evil influence breaks the bones, sucks out the marrow, drinks the blood, gnaws the intestines and the heart and devours the flesh. The invalid perishes according to the progress of this destructive work; and death speedily ensues, unless the evil genius can be driven out of it before it has committed irreparable damage. Whoever treats a sick person has therefore two equally important duties to perform. He must first discover the nature of the spirit in possession, and, if necessary, its name, and then attack it, drive it out, or even destroy it. He can only succeed by powerful magic, so he must be an expert in reciting incantations, and skilful in making amulets. He must then use medicine (drugs and diet) to contend with the disorders which the presence of the strange being has produced in the body. "(6)

(5) Maspero: Life in Ancient Egypt and Assyria, London,
1891, p. 119.

(6) Maspero: Life in Ancient Egypt and Assyria, London,
1891, p. 118.

(7) W. Wreszinski: Die Medizin der alten Aegypter, Leipzig,
J. C. Hinrichs, 1909-1912.

In this way it came about that diseases

were believed to be due to hostile spirits, or caused by the anger of a god, so that medicines, no matter how powerful, could only be expected to assuage the pain; but magic alone, incantations, spells and prayers, could remove the disease. Experience brought much of the wisdom we call empirical, and the records, extending for thousands of years, show that the Egyptians employed emetics, purgatives, enemata, diuretics, diaphoretics and even bleeding. They had a rich pharmacopoeia derived from the animal, vegetable and mineral kingdoms. In the later periods, specialism reached a remarkable development, and Herodotus remarks that the country was full of physicians;—"One treats only the diseases of the eye, another those of the head, the teeth, the abdomen, or the internal organs."

Our knowledge of Egyptian medicine is derived largely from the remarkable papyri dealing specially with this subject. Of these, six or seven are of the first importance. The most famous is that discovered by Ebers, dating from about 1500 B.C. A superb document, one of the great treasures of the Leipzig Library, it is 20.23 metres long and 30 centimetres high and in a state of wonderful preservation. Others are the Kahun, Berlin, Hearst and British Museum papyri. All these have now been published—the last three quite recently, edited by Wreszinski.(7) I show here a reproduction from which an idea may be had of these remarkable documents. They are motley collections, filled with incantations, charms, magical formulae, symbols, prayers and prescriptions for all sorts of ailments. One is impressed by the richness of the pharmacopoeia, and the high development which the art of pharmacy must have attained. There were gargles, salves, snuffs, inhalations, suppositories, fumigations, enemata, poultices and plasters; and they knew the use of opium, hemlock, the copper salts, squills and castor oil. Surgery was not very highly developed, but the knife and actual cautery were freely used. Ophthalmic surgery was practiced by specialists, and there are many prescriptions in the papyri for ophthalmia.

One department of Egyptian medicine reached a high stage of development, vis., hygiene. Cleanliness of the dwellings, of the cities and of the person was regulated by law, and the priests set a splendid example in their frequent ablutions, shaving of the entire body, and the spotless cleanliness of their clothing. As Diodorus remarks, so evenly ordered was their whole manner of life that it was as if arranged by a learned physician rather than by a lawgiver.

Two world-wide modes of practice found their earliest illustration in ancient Egypt. Magic, the first of these, represented the attitude of primitive man to nature, and really was his religion. He had no idea of immutable laws, but regarded the world about him as changeable and fickle like himself, and "to make life go as he wished, he must be able to please and propitiate or to coerce these forces outside himself."(8)

(8) L. Thorndike: The Place of Magic in the Intellectual
History of Europe, New York, 1905. p. 29.

The point of interest to us is that in the Pyramid Texts—"the oldest chapter in human thinking preserved to us, the remotest reach in the intellectual history of man which we are now able to discern"(9)—one of their six-fold contents relates to the practice of magic. A deep belief existed as to its efficacy, particularly in guiding the dead, who were said to be glorious by reason of mouths equipped with the charms, prayers and ritual of the Pyramid Texts, armed with which alone could the soul escape the innumerable dangers and ordeals of the passage through another world. Man has never lost his belief in the efficacy of magic, in the widest sense of the term. Only a very few of the most intellectual nations have escaped from its shackles. Nobody else has so clearly expressed the origins and relations of magic as Pliny in his "Natural History." "(10) 'Now, if a man consider the thing well, no marvaile it is that it hath continued thus in so great request and authoritie; for it is the onely Science which seemeth to comprise in itselfe three possessions besides, which have the command and rule of mans mind above any other whatsoever. For to begin withall, no man doubteth but that Magicke tooke root first, and proceeded from Physicke, under the presence of maintaining health, curing, and preventing diseases: things plausible to the world, crept and insinuated farther into the heart of man, with a deepe conceit of some high and divine matter therein more than ordinarie, and in comparison whereof, all other Physicke was but basely accounted. And having thus made way and entrance, the better to fortifie it selfe, and to give a goodly colour and lustre to those fair and flattering promises of things, which our nature is most given to hearken after, on goeth the habite also and cloake of religion: a point, I may tell you, that even in these daies holdeth captivate the spirit of man, and draweth away with it a greater part of the world, and nothing so much. But not content with this success and good proceeding, to gather more strength and win a greater name, shee entermingled with medicinable receipts and religious ceremonies, the skill of Astrologie and arts Mathematicall; presuming upon this, That all men by nature are very curious and desirous to know their future fortunes, and what shall betide them hereafter, persuading themselves, that all such foreknowledge dependeth upon the course and influence of the starres, which give the truest and most certain light of things to come. Being thus wholly possessed of men, and having their senses and understanding by this meanes fast ynough bound with three sure chains, no marvell if this art grew in processe of time to such an head, that it was and is at this day reputed by most nations of the earth for the paragon and cheefe of all sciences: insomuch as the mightie kings and monarchs of the Levant are altogether ruled and governed thereby."

(9) Breasted: Development of Religion and Thought in
Ancient Egypt, New York, 1912, p. 84.

(10) The Historie of the World, commonly called the Naturall
Historie of C. Plinius Secundus, translated into English by
Philemon Holland, Doctor in Physieke, London, 1601, Vol. II,
p. 371, Bk. XXX, Chap. I, Sect. 1.

The second world-wide practice which finds its earliest record among the Egyptians is the use secretions and parts of the animal body as medicine. The practice was one of great antiquity with primitive man, but the papyri already mentioned contain the earliest known records. Saliva, urine, bile, faeces, various parts of the body, dried and powdered, worms, insects, snakes were important ingredients in the pharmacopoeia. The practice became very widespread throughout the ancient world. Its extent and importance may be best gathered from chapters VII and VIII in the 28th book of Pliny's "Natural History." Several remedies are mentioned as derived from man; others from the elephant, lion, camel, crocodile, and some seventy-nine are prepared from the hyaena. The practice was widely prevalent throughout the Middle Ages, and the pharmacopoeia of the seventeenth and even of the eighteenth century contains many extraordinary ingredients. "The Royal Pharmacopoeia" of Moses Charras (London ed., 1678), the most scientific work of the day, is full of organotherapy and directions for the preparation of medicines from the most loathsome excretions. A curious thing is that with the discoveries of the mummies a belief arose as to the great efficacy of powdered mummy in various maladies. As Sir Thomas Browne remarks in his "Urn Burial": "Mummy has become merchandize. Mizraim cures wounds, and Pharaoh is sold for balsams."

One formula in everyday use has come to us in a curious way from the Egyptians. In the Osiris myth, the youthful Horus loses an eye in his battle with Set. This eye, the symbol of sacrifice, became, next to the sacred beetle, the most common talisman of the country, and all museums are rich in models of the Horus eye in glass or stone.

"When alchemy or chemistry, which had its cradle in Egypt, and derived its name from Khami, an old title for this country, passed to the hands of the Greeks, and later of the Arabs, this sign passed with it. It was also adopted to some extent by the Gnostics of the early Christian church in Egypt. In a cursive form it is found in mediaeval translations of the works of Ptolemy the astrologer, as the sign of the planet Jupiter. As such it was placed upon horoscopes and upon formula containing drugs made for administration to the body, so that the harmful properties of these drugs might be removed under the influence of the lucky planet. At present, in a slightly modified form, it still figures at the top of prescriptions written daily in Great Britain (Rx)."(11)

(11) John D. Comrie: Medicine among the Assyrians and
Egyptians in 1500 B.C., Edinburgh Medical Journal, 1909, n.
s., II, 119.

For centuries Egyptian physicians had a great reputation, and in the Odyssey (Bk. IV), Polydamna, the wife of Thonis, gives medicinal plants to Helen in Egypt—"a country producing an infinite number of drugs . . . where each physician possesses knowledge above all other men." Jeremiah (xlvi, 11) refers to the virgin daughter of Egypt, who should in vain use many medicines. Herodotus tells that Darius had at his court certain Egyptians, whom he reckoned the best skilled physicians in all the world, and he makes the interesting statement that: "Medicine is practiced among them on a plan of separation; each physician treats a single disorder, and no more: thus the country swarms with medical practitioners, some under taking to cure diseases of the eye, others of the head, others again of the teeth, others of the intestines, and some those which are not local."(12)

(12) The History of Herodotus, Blakesley's ed., Bk. II, 84.

A remarkable statement is made by Pliny, in the discussion upon the use of radishes, which are said to cure a "Phthisicke," or ulcer of the lungs—"proofe whereof was found and seen in AEgypt by occasion that the KK. there, caused dead bodies to be cut up, and anatomies to be made, for to search out the maladies whereof men died."(13)

(13) Pliny, Holland's translation, Bk. XIX, Chap. V, Sect. 26.

The study of the anatomy of mummies has thrown a very interesting light upon the diseases of the ancient Egyptians, one of the most prevalent of which appears to have been osteo-arthritis. This has been studied by Elliot Smith, Wood Jones, Ruffer and Rietti. The majority of the lesions appear to have been the common osteo-arthritis, which involved not only the men, but many of the pet animals kept in the temples. In a much higher proportion apparently than in modern days, the spinal column was involved. It is interesting to note that the "determinative" of old age in hieroglyphic writing is the picture of a man afflicted with arthritis deformans. Evidences of tuberculosis, rickets and syphilis, according to these authors, have not been found.

A study of the internal organs has been made by Ruffer, who has shown that arterio-sclerosis with calcification was a common disease 8500 years ago; and he holds that it could not have been associated with hard work or alcohol, for the ancient Egyptians did not drink spirits, and they had practically the same hours of work as modern Egyptians, with every seventh day free.

ASSYRIAN AND BABYLONIAN MEDICINE

OF equally great importance in the evolution of medicine was the practically contemporary civilization in Mesopotamia. Science here reached a much higher stage then in the valley of the Nile. An elaborate scheme of the universe was devised, a system growing out of the Divine Will, and a recognition for the first time of a law guiding and controlling heaven and earth alike. Here, too, we find medicine ancillary to religion. Disease was due to evil spirits or demons. "These 'demons'—invisible to the naked eye were the precursors of the modern 'germs' and 'microbes,' while the incantations recited by the priests are the early equivalents of the physician's prescriptions. There were different incantations for different diseases; and they were as mysterious to the masses as are the mystic formulas of the modern physician to the bewildered, yet trusting, patient. Indeed, their mysterious character added to the power supposed to reside in the incantations for driving the demons away. Medicinal remedies accompanied the recital of the incantations, but despite the considerable progress made by such nations of hoary antiquity as the Egyptians and Babylonians in the diagnosis and treatment of common diseases, leading in time to the development of an extensive pharmacology, so long as the cure of disease rested with the priests, the recital of sacred formulas, together with rites that may be conveniently grouped under the head of sympathetic magic, was regarded as equally essential with the taking of the prescribed remedies."(14)

(14) Morris Jastrow: The Liver in Antiquity and the
   Beginnings of Anatomy.
Transactions College of Physicians,
   Philadelphia, 1907, 3. s., XXIX, 117-138.

Three points of interest may be referred to in connection with Babylonian medicine. Our first recorded observations on anatomy are in connection with the art of divination—the study of the future by the interpretation of certain signs. The student recognized two divisions of divination—the involuntary, dealing with the interpretation of signs forced upon our attention, such as the phenomena of the heavens, dreams, etc., and voluntary divination, the seeking of signs, more particularly through the inspection of sacrificial animals. This method reached an extraordinary development among the Babylonians, and the cult spread to the Etruscans, Hebrews, and later to the Greeks and Romans.

Of all the organs inspected in a sacrificial animal the liver, from its size, position and richness in blood, impressed the early observers as the most important of the body. Probably on account of the richness in blood it came to be regarded as the seat of life—indeed, the seat of the soul. From this important position the liver was not dislodged for many centuries, and in the Galenic physiology it shared with the heart and the brain in the triple control of the natural, animal and vital spirits. Many expressions in literature indicate how persistent was this belief. Among the Babylonians, the word "liver" was used in hymns and other compositions precisely as we use the word "heart," and Jastrow gives a number of illustrations from Hebrew, Greek and Latin sources illustrating this usage.

The belief arose that through the inspection of this important organ in the sacrificial animal the course of future events could be predicted. "The life or soul, as the seat of life, in the sacrificial animal is, therefore, the divine element in the animal, and the god in accepting the animal, which is involved in the act of bringing it as an offering to a god, identifies himself with the animal—becomes, as it were, one with it. The life in the animal is a reflection of his own life, and since the fate of men rests with the gods, if one can succeed in entering into the mind of a god, and thus ascertain what he purposes to do, the key for the solution of the problem as to what the future has in store will have been found. The liver being the centre of vitality—the seat of the mind, therefore, as well as of the emotions—it becomes in the case of the sacrificial animal, either directly identical with the mind of the god who accepts the animal, or, at all events, a mirror in which the god's mind is reflected; or, to use another figure, a watch regulated to be in sympathetic and perfect accord with a second watch. If, therefore, one can read the liver of the sacrificial animal, one enters, as it were, into the workshop of the divine will."(15)

(15) Morris Jastrow: loc. cit., p. 122.

Hepatoscopy thus became, among the Babylonians, of extraordinary complexity, and the organ of the sheep was studied and figured as early as 3000 B.C. In the divination rites, the lobes, the gall-bladder, the appendages of the upper lobe and the markings were all inspected with unusual care. The earliest known anatomical model, which is here shown, is the clay model of a sheep's liver with the divination text dating from about 2000 B.C., from which Jastrow has worked out the modern anatomical equivalents of the Babylonian terms. To reach a decision on any point, the phenomena of the inspection of the liver were carefully recorded, and the interpretations rested on a more or less natural and original association of ideas. Thus, if the gall-bladder were swollen on the right side, it pointed to an increase in the strength of the King's army, and was favorable; if on the left side, it indicated rather success of the enemy, and was unfavorable. If the bile duct was long, it pointed to a long life. Gallstones are not infrequently mentioned in the divination texts and might be favorable, or unfavorable. Various interpretations were gathered by the scribes in the reference note-books which serve as guides for the interpretation of the omens and for text-books of instructions in the temple schools (Jastrow).

The art of divination spread widely among the neighboring nations. There are many references in the Bible to the practice. The elders of Moab and Midian came to Balaam "with the rewards of divination in their hand" (Numbers xxii, 7). Joseph's cup of divination was found in Benjamin's sack (Genesis xliv, 5, 12); and in Ezekiel (xxi, 21) the King of Babylon stood at the parting of the way and looked in the liver. Hepatoscopy was also practiced by the Etruscans, and from them it passed to the Greeks and the Romans, among whom it degenerated into a more or less meaningless form. But Jastrow states that in Babylonia and Assyria, where for several thousand years the liver was consistently employed as the sole organ of divination, there are no traces of the rite having fallen into decay, or having been abused by the priests.

In Roman times, Philostratus gives an account of the trial of Apollonius of Tyana,(16) accused of human hepatoscopy by sacrificing a boy in the practice of magic arts against the Emperor. "The liver, which the experts say is the very tripod of their art, does not consist of pure blood; for the heart retains all the uncontaminated blood, and irrigates the whole body with it by the conduits of the arteries; whereas the gall, which is situated next the liver, is stimulated by anger and depressed by fear into the hollows of the liver."

We have seen how early and how widespread was the belief in amulets and charms against the occult powers of darkness. One that has persisted with extraordinary tenacity is the belief in the Evil Eye the power of certain individuals to injure with a look. Of general belief in the older civilizations, and referred to in several places in the Bible, it passed to Greece and Rome, and today is still held fervently in many parts of Europe. The sign of "le corna,"— the first and fourth fingers extended, the others turned down and the thumb closed over them,—still used against the Evil Eye in Italy, was a mystic sign used by the Romans in the festival of Lemuralia. And we meet with the belief also in this country. A child with hemiplegia, at the Infirmary for Diseases of the Nervous System, Philadelphia, from the central part of Pennsylvania, was believed by its parents to have had the Evil Eye cast upon it.

The second contribution of Babylonia and Assyria to medicine—one that affected mankind profoundly—relates to the supposed influence of the heavenly bodies upon man's welfare. A belief that the stars in their courses fought for or against him arose early in their civilizations, and directly out of their studies on astrology and mathematics. The Macrocosm, the heavens that "declare the glory of God," reflect, as in a mirror, the Microcosm, the daily life of man on earth. The first step was the identification of the sun, moon and stars with the gods of the pantheon. Assyrian astronomical observations show an extraordinary development of practical knowledge. The movements of the sun and moon and of the planets were studied; the Assyrians knew the precession of the equinoxes and many of the fundamental laws of astronomy, and the modern nomenclature dates from their findings. In their days the signs of the zodiac corresponded practically with the twelve constellations whose names they still bear, each division being represented by the symbol of some god, as the Scorpion, the Ram, the Twins, etc. "Changes in the heavens . . . portended changes on earth. The Biblical expression 'hosts of heaven' for the starry universe admirably reflects the conception held by the Babylonian astrologers. Moon, planets and stars constituted an army in constant activity, executing military manoeuvres which were the result of deliberation and which had in view a fixed purpose. It was the function of the priest—the barqu, or 'inspector,' as the astrologer as well as the 'inspector' of the liver was called—to discover this purpose. In order to do so, a system of interpretation was evolved, less logical and less elaborate than the system of hepatoscopy, which was analyzed in the preceding chapter, but nevertheless meriting attention both as an example of the pathetic yearning of men to peer into the minds of the gods, and of the influence that Babylonian-Assyrian astrology exerted throughout the ancient world" (Jastrow).(17)

(16) Philostratus: Apollonius of Tyana, Bk. VIII, Chap.
VII, Phillimore's transl., Oxford, 1912, II, 233. See,
also, Justin: Apologies, edited by Louis Pautigny, Paris,
1904, p. 39.

(17) M. Jastrow: Aspects of Religious Belief and Practice
in Babylonia and Assyria, New York, 1911, p. 210.

With the rationalizing influence of the Persians the hold of astrology weakened, and according to Jastrow it was this, in combination with Hebrew and Greek modes of thought, that led the priests in the three centuries following the Persian occupation, to exchange their profession of diviners for that of astronomers; and this, he says, marks the beginning of the conflict between religion and science. At first an expression of primitive "science," astrology became a superstition, from which the human mind has not yet escaped. In contrast to divination, astrology does not seem to have made much impression on the Hebrews and definite references in the Bible are scanty. From Babylonia it passed to Greece (without, however, exerting any particular influence upon Greek medicine). Our own language is rich in words of astral significance derived from the Greek, e.g., disaster.

The introduction of astrology into Europe has a passing interest. Apparently the Greeks had made important advances in astronomy before coming in contact with the Babylonians,—who, in all probability, received from the former a scientific conception of the universe. "In Babylonia and Assyria we have astrology first and astronomy afterwards, in Greece we have the sequence reversed—astronomy first and astrology afterwards" (Jastrow).(18)

(18) M. Jastrow: Aspects of Religious Belief and Practice
in Babylonia and Assyria, New York, 1911, p. 256.

It is surprising to learn that, previous to their contact with the Greeks, astrology as relating to the individual—that is to say, the reading of the stars to determine the conditions under which the individual was born—had no place in the cult of the Babylonians and Assyrians. The individualistic spirit led the Greek to make his gods take note of every action in his life, and his preordained fate might be read in the stars.—"A connecting link between the individual and the movements in the heavens was found in an element which they shared in common. Both man and stars moved in obedience to forces from which there was no escape. An inexorable law controlling the planets corresponded to an equally inexorable fate ordained for every individual from his birth. Man was a part of nature and subject to its laws. The thought could therefore arise that, if the conditions in the heavens were studied under which a man was born, that man's future could be determined in accord with the beliefs associated with the position of the planets rising or visible at the time of birth or, according to other views, at the time of conception. These views take us back directly to the system of astrology developed by Babylonian baru priests. The basis on which the modified Greek system rests is likewise the same that we have observed in Babylonia—a correspondence between heaven and earth, but with this important difference, that instead of the caprice of the gods we have the unalterable fate controlling the entire universe—the movements of the heavens and the life of the individual alike" (Jastrow).(19)

(19) Ibid., pp. 257-258.

From this time on until the Renaissance, like a shadow, astrology follows astronomy. Regarded as two aspects of the same subject, the one, natural astrology, the equivalent of astronomy, was concerned with the study of the heavens, the other, judicial astrology, was concerned with the casting of horoscopes, and reading in the stars the fate of the individual.

As I mentioned, Greek science in its palmy days seems to have been very free from the bad features of astrology. Gilbert Murray remarks that "astrology fell upon the Hellenistic mind as a new disease falls upon some remote island people." But in the Greek conquest of the Roman mind, astrology took a prominent role. It came to Rome as part of the great Hellenizing movement, and the strength of its growth may be gauged from the edicts issued against astrologers as early as the middle of the second century B.C. In his introduction to his recent edition of Book II of the Astronomicon of Manilius, Garrod traces the growth of the cult, which under the Empire had an extraordinary vogue. "Though these (heavenly) signs be far removed from us, yet does he (the god) so make their influences felt, that they give to nations their life and their fate and to each man his own character. "(20) Oracles were sought on all occasions, from the planting of a tree to the mating of a horse, and the doctrine of the stars influenced deeply all phases of popular thought and religion. The professional astrologers, as Pliny(21) says, were Chaldeans, Egyptians and Greeks. The Etruscans, too, the professional diviners of Rome, cultivated the science. Many of these "Isiaci conjectores" and "astrologi de circo" were worthless charlatans, but on the whole the science seems to have attracted the attention of thoughtful men of the period. Garrod quotes the following remarkable passage from Tacitus: "My judgment wavers," he says, "I dare not say whether it be fate and necessity immutable which governs the changing course of human affairs—or just chance. Among the wisest of the ancients, as well as among their apes, you will find a conflict of opinion. Many hold fixedly the idea that our beginning and our end—that man himself—is nothing to the Gods at all. The wicked are in prosperity and the good meet tribulation. Others believe that Fate and the facts of this world work together. But this connection they trace not to planetary influences but to a concatenation of natural causes. We choose our life that is free: but the choice once made, what awaits us is fixed and ordered. Good and evil are different from the vulgar opinion of them. Often those who seem to battle with adversity are to be accounted blessed; but the many, even in their prosperity, are miserable. It needs only to bear misfortune bravely, while the fool perishes in his wealth. Outside these rival schools stands the man in the street. No one will take from him his conviction that at our birth are fixed for us the things that shall be. If some things fall out differently from what was foretold, that is due to the deceit of men that speak what they know not: calling into contempt a science to which past and present alike bear a glorious testimony" (Ann. vi, 22).

(20) Manili Astronomicon Liber II. ed. H. W. Garrod, Oxford, 1911, p. lxix, and II, ll. 84-86.

(21) Pliny: Natural History, Bk. XVIII, Chap. XXV, Sect. 57.

Cato waged war on the Greek physicians and forbade "his uilicus all resort to haruspicem, augurem, hariolum Chaldaeum," but in vain; so widespread became the belief that the great philosopher, Panaetius (who died about 111 B. C.), and two of his friends alone among the stoics, rejected the claims of astrology as a science (Garrod). So closely related was the subject of mathematics that it, too, fell into disfavor, and in the Theodosian code sentence of death was passed upon mathematicians. Long into the Middle Ages, the same unholy alliance with astrology and divination caused mathematics to be regarded with suspicion, and even Abelard calls it a nefarious study.

The third important feature in Babylonian medicine is the evidence afforded by the famous Hammurabi Code (circa 2000 B.C.)—a body of laws, civil and religious, many of which relate to the medical profession. This extraordinary document is a black diorite block 8 feet high, once containing 21 columns on the obverse, 16 and 28 columns on the reverse, with 2540 lines of writing of which now 1114 remain, and surmounted by the figure of the king receiving the law from the Sun-god. Copies of this were set up in Babylon "that anyone oppressed or injured, who had a tale of woe to tell, might come and stand before his image, that of a king of righteousness, and there read the priceless orders of the King, and from the written monument solve his problem" (Jastrow). From the enactments of the code we gather that the medical profession must have been in a highly organized state, for not only was practice regulated in detail, but a scale of fees was laid down, and penalties exacted for malpraxis. Operations were performed, and the veterinary art was recognized. An interesting feature, from which it is lucky that we have in these days escaped, is the application of the "lex talionis"—an eye for an eye, bone for a bone, and tooth for a tooth, which is a striking feature of the code.

Some of the laws of the code may be quoted:

Paragraph 215. If a doctor has treated a gentleman for a severe wound with a bronze lances and has cured the man, or has opened an abscess of the eye for a gentleman with the bronze lances and has cured the eye of the gentleman, he shall take ten shekels of silver.

218. If the doctor has treated a gentleman for a severe wound with a lances of bronze and has caused the gentleman to die, or has opened an abscess of the eye for a gentleman and has caused the loss of the gentleman's eye, one shall cut off his hands.

219. If a doctor has treated the severe wound of a slave of a poor man with a bronze lances and has caused his death, he shall render slave for slave.

220. If he has opened his abscess with a bronze lances and has made him lose his eye, he shall pay money, half his price.

221. If a doctor has cured the shattered limb of a gentleman, or has cured the diseased bowel, the patient shall give five shekels of silver to the doctor.

224. If a cow doctor or a sheep doctor has treated a cow or a sheep for a severe wound and cured it, the owner of the cow or sheep shall give one-sixth of a shekel of silver to the doctor as his fee. (22)

(22) The Oldest Code of Laws in the World; translated by C.
H. W. Johns, Edinburgh, 1903.

HEBREW MEDICINE

THE medicine of the Old Testament betrays both Egyptian and Babylonian influences; the social hygiene is a reflex of regulations the origin of which may be traced in the Pyramid Texts and in the papyri. The regulations in the Pentateuch codes revert in part to primitive times, in part represent advanced views of hygiene. There are doubts if the Pentateuch code really goes back to the days of Moses, but certainly someone "learned in the wisdom of the Egyptians" drew it up. As Neuburger briefly summarizes:

"The commands concern prophylaxis and suppression of epidemics, suppression of venereal disease and prostitution, care of the skin, baths, food, housing and clothing, regulation of labour, sexual life, discipline of the people, etc. Many of these commands, such as Sabbath rest, circumcision, laws concerning food (interdiction of blood and pork), measures concerning menstruating and lying-in women and those suffering from gonorrhoea, isolation of lepers, and hygiene of the camp, are, in view of the conditions of the climate, surprisingly rational."(23)

(23) Neuburger: History of Medicine, Oxford University
Press, 1910, Vol. I, p. 38.

Divination, not very widely practiced, was borrowed, no doubt, from Babylonia. Joseph's cup was used for the purpose, and in Numbers, the elders of Balak went to Balaam with the rewards of divination in their hands. The belief in enchantments and witchcraft was universal, and the strong enactments against witches in the Old Testament made a belief in them almost imperative until more rational beliefs came into vogue in the eighteenth and nineteenth centuries.

Whatever view we may take of it, the medicine of the New Testament is full of interest. Divination is only referred to once in the Acts (xvi, 16), where a damsel is said to be possessed of a spirit of divination "which brought her masters much gain by soothsaying." There is only one mention of astrology (Acts vii, 43); there are no witches, neither are there charms or incantations. The diseases mentioned are numerous: demoniac possession, convulsions, paralysis, skin diseases,—as leprosy,—dropsy, haemorrhages, fever, fluxes, blindness and deafness. And the cure is simple usually a fiat of the Lord, rarely with a prayer, or with the use of means such as spittle. They are all miraculous, and the same power was granted to the apostles—"power against unclean spirits, to cast them out, to heal all manner of sickness and all manner of disease." And more than this, not only the blind received their sight, the lame walked, the lepers were cleansed, the deaf heard, but even the dead were raised up. No question of the mandate. He who went about doing good was a physician of the body as well as of the soul, and could the rich promises of the Gospel have been fulfilled, there would have been no need of a new dispensation of science. It may be because the children of this world have never been able to accept its hard sayings—the insistence upon poverty, upon humility, upon peace that Christianity has lost touch no less with the practice than with the principles of its Founder. Yet, all through the centuries, the Church has never wholly abandoned the claim to apostolic healing; nor is there any reason why she should. To the miraculous there should be no time limit—only conditions have changed and nowadays to have a mountain-moving faith is not easy. Still, the possession is cherished, and it adds enormously to the spice and variety of life to know that men of great intelligence, for example, my good friend, Dr. James J. Walsh of New York, believe in the miracles of Lourdes.(24) Only a few weeks ago, the Bishop of London followed with great success, it is said, the practice of St. James. It does not really concern us much—as Oriental views of disease and its cure have had very little influence on the evolution of scientific medicine—except in illustration of the persistence of an attitude towards disease always widely prevalent, and, indeed, increasing. Nor can we say that the medicine of our great colleague, St. Luke, the Beloved Physician, whose praise is in the Gospels, differs so fundamentally from that of the other writings of the New Testament that we can claim for it a scientific quality. The stories of the miracles have technical terms and are in a language adorned by medical phraseology, but the mental attitude towards disease is certainly not that of a follower of Hippocrates, nor even of a scientifically trained contemporary of Dioscorides.(25)

(24) Psychotherapy, New York, 1919, p. 79, "I am convinced
   that miracles happen there. There is more than natural power
      manifest."

(25) See Luke the Physician, by Harnack, English ed., 1907,
   and W. K. Hobart, The Medical Language of St. Luke, 1882.

CHINESE AND JAPANESE MEDICINE

CHINESE medicine illustrates the condition at which a highly intellectual people may arrive, among whom thought and speculation were restricted by religious prohibitions. Perhaps the chief interest in its study lies in the fact that we may see today the persistence of views about disease similar to those which prevailed in ancient Egypt and Babylonia. The Chinese believe in a universal animism, all parts being animated by gods and spectres, and devils swarm everywhere in numbers incalculable. The universe was spontaneously created by the operation of its Tao, "composed of two souls, the Yang and the Yin; the Yang represents light, warmth, production, and life, as also the celestial sphere from which all those blessings emanate; the Yin is darkness, cold, death, and the earth, which, unless animated by the Yang or heaven, is dark, cold, dead. The Yang and the Yin are divided into an infinite number of spirits respectively good and bad, called shen and kwei; every man and every living being contains a shen and a kwei, infused at birth, and departing at death, to return to the Yang and the Yin. Thus man with his dualistic soul is a microcosmos, born from the Macrocosmos spontaneously. Even every object is animated, as well as the Universe of which it is a part.

"(26)

(26) J. J. M. de Groot: Religious System of China, Vol. VI,
   Leyden, 1910, p. 929.

In the animistic religion of China, the Wu represented a group of persons of both sexes, who wielded, with respect to the world of spirits, capacities and powers not possessed by the rest of men. Many practitioners of Wu were physicians who, in addition to charms and enchantments, used death-banishing medicinal herbs. Of great antiquity, Wu-ism has changed in some ways its outward aspect, but has not altered its fundamental characters. The Wu, as exorcising physicians and practitioners of the medical art, may be traced in classical literature to the time of Confucius. In addition to charms and spells, there were certain famous poems which were repeated, one of which, by Han Yu, of the T'ang epoch, had an extraordinary vogue. De Groot says that the "Ling," or magical power of this poem must have been enormous, seeing that its author was a powerful mandarin, and also one of the loftiest intellects China has produced. This poetic febrifuge is translated in full by de Groot (VI, 1054-1055), and the demon of fever, potent chiefly in the autumn, is admonished to begone to the clear and limpid waters of the deep river.

In the High Medical College at Court, in the T'ang Dynasty, there were four classes of Masters, attached to its two High Medical Chiefs: Masters of Medicine, of Acupuncture, of Manipulation, and two Masters for Frustration by means of Spells.

Soothsaying and exorcism may be traced far back to the fifth and sixth centuries B.C.

In times of epidemic the specialists of Wu-ism, who act as seers, soothsayers and exorcists, engage in processions, stripped to the waist, dancing in a frantic, delirious state, covering themselves with blood by means of prick-balls, or with needles thrust through their tongues, or sitting or stretching themselves on nail points or rows of sword edges. In this way they frighten the spectres of disease. They are nearly all young, and are spoken of as 'divining youths," and they use an exorcising magic based on the principle that legions of spectres prone to evil live in the machine of the world. (De Groot, VI, 983-985.)

The Chinese believe that it is the Tao, or "Order of the Universe," which affords immunity from evil, and according to whether or no the birth occurred in a beneficent year, dominated by four double cyclical characters, the horoscope is "heavy" or "light." Those with light horoscopes are specially prone to incurable complaints, but much harm can be averted if such an individual be surrounded with exorcising objects, if he be given proper amulets to wear and proper medicines to swallow, and by selecting for him auspicious days and hours.

Two or three special points may be referred to. The doctrine of the pulse reached such extraordinary development that the whole practice of the art centred round its different characters. There were scores of varieties, which in complication and detail put to confusion the complicated system of some of the old Graeco-Roman writers. The basic idea seems to have been that each part and organ had its own proper pulse, and just as in a stringed instrument each chord has its own tone, so in the human body, if the pulses were in harmony, it meant health; if there was discord, it meant disease. These Chinese views reached Europe in the seventeenth and eighteenth centuries, and there is a very elaborate description of them in Floyer's well-known book.(27) And the idea of harmony in the pulse is met with into the eighteenth century.

(27) Sir John Floyer: The Physician's Pulse Watch, etc.,
   London, 1707.

Organotherapy was as extensively practiced in China as in Egypt. Parts of organs, various secretions and excretions are very commonly used. One useful method of practice reached a remarkable development, viz., the art of acupuncture—the thrusting of fine needles more or less deeply into the affected part. There are some 388 spots on the body in which acupuncture could be performed, and so well had long experience taught them as to the points of danger, that the course of the arteries may be traced by the tracts that are avoided. The Chinese practiced inoculation for smallpox as early as the eleventh century.

Even the briefest sketch of the condition of Chinese medicine leaves the impression of the appalling stagnation and sterility that may afflict a really intelligent people for thousands of years. It is doubtful if they are today in a very much more advanced condition than were the Egyptians at the time when the Ebers Papyrus was written. From one point of view it is an interesting experiment, as illustrating the state in which a people may remain who have no knowledge of anatomy, physiology or pathology.

Early Japanese medicine has not much to distinguish it from the Chinese. At first purely theurgic, the practice was later characterized by acupuncture and a refined study of the pulse. It has an extensive literature, largely based upon the Chinese, and extending as far back as the beginning of the Christian era. European medicine was introduced by the Portuguese and the Dutch, whose "factory" or "company" physicians were not without influence upon practice. An extraordinary stimulus was given to the belief in European medicine by a dissection made by Mayeno in 1771 demonstrating the position of the organs as shown in the European anatomical tables, and proving the Chinese figures to be incorrect. The next day a translation into Japanese of the anatomical work of Kulmus was begun, and from its appearance in 1773 may be dated the commencement of reforms in medicine. In 1793, the work of de Gorter on internal medicine was translated, and it is interesting to know that before the so-called "opening of Japan" many European works on medicine had been published. In 1857, a Dutch medical school was started in Yedo. Since the political upheaval in 1868, Japan has made rapid progress in scientific medicine, and its institutions and teachers are now among the best known in the world.(28)

(28) See Y. Fujikawa, Geschichte der Medizin in Japan,
Tokyo, 1911.

CHAPTER II — GREEK MEDICINE

OGRAIAE gentis decus! let us sing with Lucretius, one of the great interpreters of Greek thought. How grand and how true is his paean!

Out of the night, out of the blinding night
Thy beacon flashes;—hail, beloved light
Of Greece and Grecian; hail, for in the mirk
Thou cost reveal each valley and each height.

Thou art my leader, and the footprints shine,
Wherein I plant my own.

The world was shine to read, and having read,
Before thy children's eyes thou didst outspread
The fruitful page of knowledge, all the wealth
Of wisdom, all her plenty for their bread.

(Bk. III.—Translated by D. A. Slater.)

Let us come out of the murky night of the East, heavy with
phantoms,
into the bright daylight of the West, into the company of men
whose
thoughts made our thoughts, and whose ways made our ways—the men
who first dared to look on nature with the clear eyes of the
mind.

Browning's famous poem, "Childe Roland to the Dark Tower Came," is an allegory of the pilgrimage of man through the dark places of the earth, on a dismal path beset with demons, and strewn with the wreckage of generations of failures. In his ear tolled the knell of all the lost adventurers, his peers, all lost, lost within sight of the dark Tower itself—

The round squat turret, blind as the fool's heart,
Built of brown stone, without a counterpart
In the whole world.

lost in despair at an all-encircling mystery. Not so the Greek Childe Roland who set the slug-horn to his lips and blew a challenge. Neither Shakespeare nor Browning tells us what happened, and the old legend, Childe Roland, is the incarnation of the Greek spirit, the young, light-hearted master of the modern world, at whose trumpet blast the dark towers of ignorance, superstition and deceit have vanished into thin air, as the baseless fabric of a dream. Not that the jeering phantoms have flown! They still beset, in varied form, the path of each generation; but the Achaian Childe Roland gave to man self-confidence, and taught him the lesson that nature's mysteries, to be solved, must be challenged. On a portal of one of the temples of Isis in Egypt was carved: "I am whatever hath been, is, or ever will be, and my veil no man has yet lifted."

The veil of nature the Greek lifted and herein lies his value to us. What of this Genius? How did it arise among the peoples of the AEgean Sea? Those who wish to know the rock whence science was hewn may read the story told in vivid language by Professor Gomperz in his "Greek Thinkers," the fourth volume of which has recently been published (Murray, 1912; Scribner, 1912). In 1912, there was published a book by one of the younger Oxford teachers, "The Greek Genius and Its Meaning to Us,"(1) from which those who shrink from the serious study of Gomperz' four volumes may learn something of the spirit of Greece. Let me quote a few lines from his introduction:

(1) By R. W. Livingstone, Clarendon Press, Oxford, 1912 (2d ed., revised, 1915).

"Europe has nearly four million square miles; Lancashire has 1,700; Attica has 700. Yet this tiny country has given us an art which we, with it and all that the world has done since it for our models, have equalled perhaps, but not surpassed. It has given us the staple of our vocabulary in every domain of thought and knowledge. Politics, tyranny, democracy, anarchism, philosophy, physiology, geology, history—these are all Greek words. It has seized and up to the present day kept hold of our higher education. It has exercised an unfailing fascination, even on minds alien or hostile. Rome took her culture thence. Young Romans completed their education in the Greek schools. And so it was with natures less akin to Greece than the Roman. St. Paul, a Hebrew of the Hebrews, who called the wisdom of the Greeks foolishness, was drawn to their Areopagus, and found himself accommodating his gospel to the style, and quoting verses from the poets of this alien race. After him, the Church, which was born to protest against Hellenism, translated its dogmas into the language of Greek thought and finally crystallized them in the philosophy of Aristotle."

Whether a plaything of the gods or a cog in the wheels of the universe this was the problem which life offered to the thinking Greek; and in undertaking its solution, he set in motion the forces that have made our modern civilization. That the problem remains unsolved is nothing in comparison with the supreme fact that in wrestling with it, and in studying the laws of the machine, man is learning to control the small section of it with which he is specially concerned. The veil of thaumaturgy which shrouded the Orient, while not removed, was rent in twain, and for the first time in history, man had a clear vision of the world about him—"had gazed on Nature's naked loveliness" ("Adonais") unabashed and unaffrighted by the supernatural powers about him. Not that the Greek got rid of his gods—far from it!—but he made them so like himself, and lived on terms of such familiarity with them that they inspired no terror.(2)

(2) "They made deities in their own image, in the likeness
of an image of corruptible man. Sua cuique deu fit dira
cupido. 'Each man's fearful passion becomes his god.' Yes,
and not passions only, but every impulse, every aspiration,
every humour, every virtue, every whim. In each of his
activities the Greek found something wonderful, and called
it God: the hearth at which he warmed himself and cooked his
food, the street in which his house stood, the horse he
rode, the cattle he pastured, the wife he married, the child
that was born to him, the plague of which he died or from
which he recovered, each suggested a deity, and he made one
to preside over each. So too with qualities and powers more
abstract." R.W. Livingstone: The Greek Genius and Its
Meaning to Us, pp. 51-52.

Livingstone discusses the Greek Genius as displayed to us in certain "notes"—the Note of Beauty—the Desire for Freedom—the Note of Directness—the Note of Humanism—the Note of Sanity and of Many-sidedness. Upon some of these characteristics we shall have occasion to dwell in the brief sketch of the rise of scientific medicine among this wonderful people.

We have seen that the primitive man and in the great civilizations of Egypt and Babylonia, the physician evolved from the priest—in Greece he had a dual origin, philosophy and religion. Let us first trace the origins in the philosophers, particularly in the group known as the Ionian Physiologists, whether at home or as colonists in the south of Italy, in whose work the beginnings of scientific medicine may be found. Let me quote a statement from Gomperz:

"We can trace the springs of Greek success achieved and maintained by the great men of Hellas on the field of scientific inquiry to a remarkable conjunction of natural gifts and conditions. There was the teeming wealth of constructive imagination united with the sleepless critical spirit which shrank from no test of audacity; there was the most powerful impulse to generalization coupled with the sharpest faculty for descrying and distinguishing the finest shades of phenomenal peculiarity, there was the religion of Hellas, which afforded complete satisfaction to the requirements of sentiment, and yet left the intelligence free to perform its destructive work; there were the political conditions of a number of rival centres of intellect, of a friction of forces, excluding the possibility of stagnation, and, finally, of an order of state and society strict enough to curb the excesses of 'children crying for the moon,' and elastic enough not to hamper the soaring flight of superior minds. We have already made acquaintance with two of the sources from which the spirit of criticism derived its nourishment—the metaphysical and dialectical discussions practiced by the Eleatic philosophers, and the semi-historical method which was applied to the myths by Hecataeus and Herodotus. A third source is to be traced to the schools of the physicians. These aimed at eliminating the arbitrary element from the view and knowledge of nature, the beginnings of which were bound up with it in a greater or less degree, though practically without exception and by the force of an inner necessity. A knowledge of medicine was destined to correct that defect, and we shall mark the growth of its most precious fruits in the increased power of observation and the counterpoise it offered to hasty generalizations, as well as in the confidence which learnt to reject untenable fictions, whether produced by luxuriant imagination or by a priori speculations, on the similar ground of self-reliant sense-perception."(3)

(3) Gomperz: Greek Thinkers, Vol. I, p. 276.

The nature philosophers of the Ionian days did not contribute much to medicine proper, but their spirit and their outlook upon nature influenced its students profoundly. Their bold generalizations on the nature of matter and of the elements are still the wonder of chemists. We may trace to one of them, Anaximenes, who regarded air as the primary principle, the doctrine of the "pneuma," or the breath of life—the psychic force which animates the body and leaves it at death—"Our soul being air, holds us together." Of another, the famous Heraclitus, possibly a physician, the existing fragments do not relate specially to medicine; but to the philosopher of fire may be traced the doctrine of heat and moisture, and their antitheses, which influenced practice for many centuries. There is evidence in the Hippocratic treatise peri sarkwn of an attempt to apply this doctrine to the human body. The famous expression, panta rhei,—"all things are flowing,"—expresses the incessant flux in which he believed and in which we know all matter exists. No one has said a ruder thing of the profession, for an extant fragment reads: ". . . physicians, who cut, burn, stab, and rack the sick, then complain that they do not get any adequate recompense for it."(4)

(4) J. Burnet: Early Greek Philosophy, 1892, p. 137,
Bywater's no. LVIII.

The South Italian nature philosophers contributed much more to the science of medicine, and in certain of the colonial towns there were medical schools as early as the fifth century B.C. The most famous of these physician philosophers was Pythagoras, whose life and work had an extraordinary influence upon medicine, particularly in connection with his theory of numbers, and the importance of critical days. His discovery of the dependence of the pitch of sound on the length of the vibrating chord is one of the most fundamental in acoustics. Among the members of the school which he founded at Crotona were many physicians. who carried his views far and wide throughout Magna Graecia. Nothing in his teaching dominated medicine so much as the doctrine of numbers, the sacredness of which seems to have had an enduring fascination for the medical mind. Many of the common diseases, such as malaria, or typhus, terminating abruptly on special days, favored this belief. How dominant it became and how persistent you may judge from the literature upon critical days, which is rich to the middle of the eighteenth century.

One member of the Crotonian school, Alcmaeon, achieved great distinction in both anatomy and physiology. He first recognized the brain as the organ of the mind, and made careful dissections of the nerves, which he traced to the brain. He described the optic nerves and the Eustachian tubes, made correct observations upon vision, and refuted the common view that the sperma came from the spinal cord. He suggested the definition of health as the maintenance of equilibrium, or an "isonomy" in the material qualities of the body. Of all the South Italian physicians of this period, the personality of none stands out in stronger outlines than that of Empedocles of Agrigentum—physician, physiologist, religious teacher, politician and poet. A wonder-worker, also, and magician, he was acclaimed in the cities as an immortal god by countless thousands desiring oracles or begging the word of healing. That he was a keen student of nature is witnessed by many recorded observations in anatomy and physiology; he reasoned that sensations travel by definite paths to the brain. But our attention must be confined to his introduction of the theory of the four elements—fire, air, earth and water—of which, in varying quantities, all bodies were made up. Health depended upon the due equilibrium of these primitive substances; disease was their disturbance. Corresponding to those were the four essential qualities of heat and cold, moisture and dryness, and upon this four-fold division was engrafted by the later physicians the doctrine of the humors which, from the days of Hippocrates almost to our own, dominated medicine. All sorts of magical powers were attributed to Empedocles. The story of Pantheia whom he called back to life after a thirty days' trance has long clung in the imagination. You remember how Matthew Arnold describes him in the well-known poem, "Empedocles on Etna"—

But his power
Swells with the swelling evil of this time,
And holds men mute to see where it will rise.
He could stay swift diseases in old days,
Chain madmen by the music of his lyre,
Cleanse to sweet airs the breath of poisonous streams,
And in the mountain-chinks inter the winds.
This he could do of old—(5)

a quotation which will give you an idea of some of the powers attributed to this wonder-working physician.

(5) Poetical Works of Matthew Arnold, Macmillan & Co., 1898,
p. 440.

But of no one of the men of this remarkable circle have we such definite information as of the Crotonian physician Democedes, whose story is given at length by Herodotus; and his story has also the great importance of showing that, even at this early period, a well-devised scheme of public medical service existed in the Greek cities. It dates from the second half of the sixth century B.C.—fully two generations before Hippocrates. A Crotonian, Democedes by name, was found among the slaves of Oroetes. Of his fame as a physician someone had heard and he was called in to treat the dislocated ankle of King Darius. The wily Greek, longing for his home, feared that if he confessed to a knowledge of medicine there would be no chance of escape, but under threat of torture he undertook a treatment which proved successful.

Then Herodotus tells his story—how, ill treated at home in Crotona, Democedes went to AEgina, where he set up as a physician and in the second year the State of AEgina hired his services at the price of a talent. In the third year, the Athenians engaged him at 100 minae; and in the fourth, Polycrates of Samos at two talents. Democedes shared the misfortunes of Polycrates and was taken prisoner by Oroetes. Then Herodotus tells how he cured Atossa, the daughter of Cyrus and wife of Darius, of a severe abscess of the breast, but on condition that she help him to escape, and she induced her husband to send an expedition of exploration to Greece under the guidance of Democedes, but with the instructions at all costs to bring back the much prized physician. From Tarentum, Democedes escaped to his native city, but the Persians followed him, and it was with the greatest difficulty that he escaped from their hands. Deprived of their guide, the Persians gave up the expedition and sailed for Asia. In palliation of his flight, Democedes sent a message to Darius that he was engaged to the daughter of Milo, the wrestler, who was in high repute with the King. (6)

(6) The well-known editor of Herodotus, R. W. Macan, Master
  of University College, Oxford, in his Hellenikon. A Sheaf
  of Sonnets after Herodotus (Oxford, 1898) has included a
  poem which may be quoted in connection with this incident:

  NOSTALGY
  Atossa, child of Cyrus king of kings,
    healed by Greek science of a morbid breast,
    gave lord Dareios neither love nor rest
    till he fulfilled her vain imaginings.
  "Sir, show our Persian folk your sceptre's wings!
    Enlarge my sire's and brother's large bequest.
    This learned Greek shall guide your galleys west,
    and Dorian slave-girls grace our banquetings."

So said she, taught of that o'erartful man,
  the Italiote captive, Kroton's Demokede,
  who recked not what of maladies began,
  nor who in Asia and in Greece might bleed,
  if he—so writes the guileless Thurian—
  regained his home, and freedom of the Mede.

Plato has several references to these state physicians, who were evidently elected by a public assembly: "When the assembly meets to elect a physician,' and the office was yearly, for in "The Statesman" we find the following:(7) "When the year of office has expired, the pilot, or physician has to come before a court of review" to answer any charges. The physician must have been in practice for some time and attained eminence, before he was deemed worthy of the post of state physician.

(7) Jowett: Dialogues of Plato, 3d ed., Statesman, Vol. IV,
  p. 502 (Stephanus, II, 298 E)

"If you and I were physicians, and were advising one another that we were competent to practice as state-physicians, should I not ask about you, and would you not ask about me, Well, but how about Socrates himself, has he good health? and was anyone else ever known to be cured by him whether slave or freeman?"(7a)

(7a) Jowett: Dialogues of Plato, 3d ed., Gorgias, Vol. II,
  p. 407 (Stephanus, I, 514 D).

All that is known of these state physicians has been collected by Pohl,(8) who has traced their evolution into Roman times. That they were secular, independent of the AEsculapian temples, that they were well paid, that there was keen competition to get the most distinguished men, that they were paid by a special tax and that they were much esteemed—are facts to be gleaned from Herodotus and from the inscriptions. The lapidary records, extending over 1000 years, collected by Professor Oehler(8a) of Reina, throw an important light on the state of medicine in Greece and Rome. Greek vases give representations of these state doctors at work. Dr. E. Pottier has published one showing the treatment of a patient in the clinic.(8b)

(8) R. Pohl: De Graecorum medicis publicis, Berolini,
  Reimer, 1905; also Janus, Harlem, 1905, X, 491-494.

(8a) J Oehler: Janus, Harlem, 1909, XIV, 4; 111.

(8b) E. Pottier: Une clinique grecque au Ve siecle,
  Monuments et Memoires, XIII, p. 149. Paris, 1906 (Fondation
  Eugene Piot).

That dissections were practiced by this group of nature philosophers is shown not only by the studies of Alcmaeon, but we have evidence that one of the latest of them, Diogenes of Apollonia, must have made elaborate dissections. In the "Historia Animalium"(9) of Aristotle occurs his account of the blood vessels, which is by far the most elaborate met with in the literature until the writings of Galen. It has, too, the great merit of accuracy (if we bear in mind the fact that it was not until after Aristotle that arteries and veins were differentiated), and indications are given as to the vessels from which blood may be drawn.

(9) The Works of Aristotle, Oxford, Clarendon Press, Vol.
  IV, 1910, Bk. III, Chaps. II-IV, pp. 511b-515b.

ASKLEPIOS

No god made with hands, to use the scriptural phrase, had a more successful "run" than Asklepios—for more than a thousand years the consoler and healer of the sons of men. Shorn of his divine attributes he remains our patron saint, our emblematic God of Healing, whose figure with the serpents appears in our seals and charters. He was originally a Thessalian chieftain, whose sons, Machaon and Podalirius, became famous physicians and fought in the Trojan War. Nestor, you may remember, carried off the former, declaring, in the oft-quoted phrase, that a doctor was better worth saving than many warriors unskilled in the treatment of wounds. Later genealogies trace his origin to Apollo,(10) as whose son he is usually regarded. "In the wake of northern tribes this god Aesculapius—a more majestic figure than the blameless leech of Homer's song—came by land to Epidaurus and was carried by sea to the east-ward island of Cos. Aesculapius grew in importance with the growth of Greece, but may not have attained his greatest power until Greece and Rome were one."(11)

(10) W. H. Roscher: Lexikon der griechischen und romischen
　Mythologie, Leipzig, 1886, I, p. 624.

(11) Louis Dyer: Studies of the Gods in Greece, 1891, p.
　221.

A word on the idea of the serpent as an emblem of the healing art which goes far back into antiquity. The mystical character of the snake, and the natural dread and awe inspired by it, early made it a symbol of supernatural power. There is a libation vase of Gudea, c. 2350 B.C., found at Telloh, now in the Louvre (probably the earliest representation of the symbol), with two serpents entwined round a staff (Jastrow, Pl. 4). From the earliest times the snake has been associated with mystic and magic power, and even today, among native races, it plays a part in the initiation of medicine men.

In Greece, the serpent became a symbol of Apollo, and prophetic serpents were kept and fed at his shrine, as well as at that of his son, Asklepios. There was an idea, too, that snakes had a knowledge of herbs, which is referred to in the famous poem of Nikander on Theriaka.(12) You may remember that when Alexander, the famous quack and oracle monger, depicted by Lucian, started out "for revenue," the first thing he did was to provide himself with two of the large, harmless, yellow snakes of Asia Minor.

(12) Lines 31, etc., and Scholia; cf. W. R. Halliday: Greek
　Divination, London, 1913, p. 88.

The exact date of the introduction of the cult into Greece is not known, but its great centres were at Epidaurus, Cos, Pergamos and Tricca. It throve with wonderful rapidity. Asklepios became one of the most popular of the gods. By the time of Alexander it is estimated that there were between three and four hundred temples dedicated to him.

His worship was introduced into Rome at the time of the Great Plague at the beginning of the third century B. C. (as told by Livy in Book XI), and the temple on the island of Tiber became a famous resort. If you can transfer in imagination the Hot Springs of Virginia to the neighborhood of Washington, and put there a group of buildings such as are represented in these outlines of Caton's(13) (p. 52), add a sumptuous theatre with seating capacity for 20,000, a stadium 600 feet long with a seating capacity of 12,000, and all possible accessories of art and science, you will have an idea of what the temple at Epidaurus, a few miles from Athens, was. "The cult flourished mostly in places which, through climatic or hygienic advantages, were natural health resorts. Those favoured spots on hill or mountain, in the shelter of forests, by rivers or springs of pure flowing water, were conducive to health. The vivifying air, the well cultivated gardens surrounding the shrine, the magnificent view, all tended to cheer the heart with new hope of cure. Many of these temples owed their fame to mineral or merely hot springs. To the homely altars, erected originally by sacred fountains in the neighbourhood of health-giving mineral springs, were later added magnificent temples, pleasure-grounds for festivals, gymnasia in which bodily ailments were treated by physical exercises, baths and inunctions, also, as is proved by excavations, living rooms for the patients. Access to the shrine was forbidden to the unclean and the impure, pregnant women and the mortally afflicted were kept away; no dead body could find a resting-place within the holy precincts, the shelter and the cure of the sick being undertaken by the keepers of inns and boarding-houses in the neighbourhood. The suppliants for aid had to submit to careful purification, to bathe in sea, river or spring, to fast for a prescribed time, to abjure wine and certain articles of diet, and they were only permitted to enter the temple when they were adequately prepared by cleansing, inunction and fumigation. This lengthy and exhausting preparation, partly dietetic, partly suggestive, was accompanied by a solemn service of prayer and sacrifice, whose symbolism tended highly to excite the imagination."(14)

(13) Caton: Temples and Ritual of Asklepios, 2d ed.,
　London, 1900.

(14) Max Neuburger: History of Medicine, English
　translation, Oxford, 1910, p. 94.

The temples were in charge of members of the guild or fraternity, the head of which was often, though not necessarily, a physician. The Chief was appointed annually. From Caton's excellent sketch(15) you can get a good idea of the ritual, but still better is the delightful description given in the "Plutus" of Aristophanes. After offering honey-cakes and baked meats on the altar, the suppliants arranged themselves on the pallets.

(15) Caton: Temples and Ritual of Asklepios, 2d ed.,
　London, 1900.

　Soon the Temple servitor
　Put out the lights and bade us fall asleep,

Nor stir, nor speak, whatever noise we heard.
So down we lay in orderly repose.
And I could catch no slumber, not one wink,
Struck by a nice tureen of broth which stood
A little distance from an old wife's head,
Whereto I marvellously longed to creep.
Then, glancing upwards, I beheld the priest
Whipping the cheese-cakes and figs from off
The holy table; thence he coasted round
To every altar spying what was left.
And everything he found he consecrated
Into a sort of sack—(16)

a procedure which reminds one of the story of "Bel and the Dragon." Then the god came, in the person of the priest, and scanned each patient. He did not neglect physical measures, as he brayed in a mortar cloves, Tenian garlic, verjuice, squills and Sphettian vinegar, with which he made application to the eyes of the patient.

(16) Aristophanes: B. B. Roger's translation, London, Bell
& Sons, 1907, Vol. VI, ll. 668, etc., 732 ff.

Then the God clucked,
And out there issued from the holy shrine
Two great, enormous serpents.
And underneath the scarlet cloth they crept,
And licked his eyelids, as it seemed to me;
And, mistress dear, before you could have drunk
Of wine ten goblets, Wealth arose and saw.(17)

(17) Ibid.

The incubation sleep, in which indications of cure were divinely sent, formed an important part of the ritual.

The Asklepieion, or Health Temple of Cos, recently excavated, is of special interest, as being at the birthplace of Hippocrates, who was himself an Asklepiad. It is known that Cos was a great medical school. The investigations of Professor Rudolf Hertzog have shown that this temple was very nearly the counterpart of the temple at Epidaurus.

The AEsculapian temples may have furnished a rare field for empirical enquiry. As with our modern hospitals, the larger temple had rich libraries, full of valuable manuscripts and records of cases. That there may have been secular Asklepiads connected with the temple, who were freed entirely from its superstitious practices and theurgic rites, is regarded as doubtful; yet is perhaps not so doubtful as one might think. How often have we physicians to bow ourselves in the house of Rimmon! It is very much the same today at Lourdes, where lay physicians have to look after scores of patients whose faith is too weak or whose maladies are too strong to be relieved by Our Lady of this famous shrine. Even in the Christian era, there is evidence of the association of distinguished physicians with AEsculapian temples. I notice that in one of his anatomical treatises, Galen speaks with affection of a citizen of Pergamos who has been a great benefactor of the AEsculapian temple of that city. In "Marius, the Epicurean," Pater gives a delightful sketch of one of those temple health resorts, and brings in Galen, stating that he had himself undergone the temple sleep; but to this I can find no reference in the general index of Galen's works.

From the votive tablets found at Epidaurus, we get a very good idea of the nature of the cases and of the cures. A large number of them have now been deciphered. There are evidences of various forms of diseases of the joints, affections of women, wounds, baldness, gout; but we are again in the world of miracles, as you may judge from the following: "Heraicus of Mytilene is bald and entreats the God to make his hair grow. An ointment is applied over night and the next morning he has a thick crop of hair."

There are indications that operations were performed and abscesses opened. From one we gather that dropsy was treated in a novel way: Asklepios cuts off the patient's head, holds him up by the heels, lets the water run out, claps on the patient's head again. Here is one of the invocations: "Oh, blessed Asklepios, God of Healing, it is thanks to thy skill that Diophantes hopes to be relieved from his incurable and horrible gout, no longer to move like a crab, no longer to walk upon thorns, but to have sound feet as thou hast decreed."

The priests did not neglect the natural means of healing. The inscriptions show that great attention was paid to diet, exercise, massage and bathing, and that when necessary, drugs were used. Birth and death were believed to defile the sacred precincts, and it was not until the time of the Antonines that provision was made at Epidaurus for these contingencies.

One practice of the temple was of special interest, viz., the incubation sleep, in which dreams were suggested to the patients. In the religion of Babylonia, an important part was played by the mystery of sleep, and the interpretation of dreams; and no doubt from the East the Greeks took over the practice of divination in sleep, for in the AEsculapian cult also, the incubation sleep played a most important role. That it continued in later times is well indicated in the orations of Aristides, the arch-neurasthenic of ancient history, who was a great dreamer of dreams. The oracle of Amphiaraus in Attica sent dreams into the hearts of his consultants. "The priests take the inquirer, and keep him fasting from food for one day, and from wine for three days, to give him perfect spiritual lucidity to absorb the divine communication" (Phillimore's "Apollonius of Tyana," Bk. II, Ch. XXXVII) How incubation sleep was carried into the Christian Church, its association with St. Cosmas and St. Damian and other saints, its practice throughout the Middle Ages, and its continuation to our own time may be read in the careful study of the subject made by Miss Hamilton (now Mrs. Dickens).(18)

There are still in parts of Greece and in Asia Minor shrines at which incubation is practiced regularly, and if one may judge from the reports, with as great success as in Epidaurus. At one place in Britain, Christchurch in Monmouthshire, incubation was carried on till the early part of the nineteenth century. Now the profession has come back to the study of dreams,(19) and there are professors as ready to give suggestive interpretations to them, as in the days of Aristides. As usual, Aristotle seems to have said the last word on the subject: "Even scientific physicians tell us that one should pay diligent attention to dreams, and to hold this view is reasonable also for those who are not practitioners but speculative philosophers,"(20) but it is asking too much to think that the Deity would trouble to send dreams to very simple people and to animals, if they were designed in any way to reveal the future.

In its struggle with Christianity, Paganism made its last stand in the temples of Asklepios. The miraculous healing of the saints superseded the cures of the heathen god, and it was wise to adopt the useful practice of his temple.

(18) Mary Hamilton: Incubation, or the Cure of Disease in
Pagan Temples and Christian Churches, London, 1906.

(19) Freud: The Interpretation of Dreams, translation of
third edition by A. A. Brill, 1913.

(20) Aristotle: Parva Naturalia, De divinatione per
somnium, Ch. I, Oxford ed., Vol. III, 463 a.

HIPPOCRATES AND THE HIPPOCRATIC WRITINGS

DESERVEDLY the foundation of Greek Medicine is associated with the name of Hippocrates, a native of the island of Cos; and yet he is a shadowy personality, about whom we have little accurate first-hand information. This is in strong contrast to some of his distinguished contemporaries and successors, for example, Plato and Aristotle, about whom we have such full and accurate knowledge. You will, perhaps, be surprised to hear that the only contemporary mention of Hippocrates is made by Plato. In the "Protagoras," the young Hippocrates, son of Apollodorus has come to Protagoras, "that mighty wise man," to learn the science and knowledge of human life. Socrates asked him: "If . . . you had thought of going to Hippocrates of Cos, the Asclepiad, and were about to give him your money, and some one had said to you, 'You are paying money to your namesake Hippocrates, O Hippocrates; tell me, what is he that you give him money?' how would you have answered?" "I should say," he replied, "that I gave money to him as a physician." "And what will he make of you?" "A physician," he said. And in the Phaedrus, in reply to a question of Socrates whether the nature of the soul could be known intelligently without knowing the nature of the whole, Phaedrus replies: "Hippocrates, the Asclepiad, says that the nature, even of the body, can only be understood as a whole." (Plato, I, 311; III, 270—Jowett, I, 131, 479.)

Several lives of Hippocrates have been written. The one most frequently quoted is that of Soranus of Ephesus (not the famous physician of the time of Trajan), and the statements which he gives are usually accepted, viz., that he was born in the island of Cos in the year 460 B.C.; that he belonged to an Asklepiad family of distinction, that he travelled extensively, visiting Thrace, Thessaly, and various other parts of Greece; that he returned to Cos, where he became the most renowned physician of his period, and died about 375 B.C. Aristotle mentions him but once, calling him "the great Hippocrates." Busts of him are common; one of the earliest of which, and I am told the best, dating from Roman days and now in the British Museum, is here represented.

Of the numerous writings attributed to Hippocrates it cannot easily be determined which are really the work of the Father of Medicine himself. They were collected at the time of the Alexandrian School, and it became customary to write commentaries upon them; much of the most important information we have about them, we derive from Galen. The earliest manuscript is the "Codex Laurentianus" of Florence, dating from the ninth century, a specimen page of which (thanks to Commendatore Biagi) is annexed. Those of you who are interested, and wish to have full references to the various works attributed to Hippocrates, will find them in "Die Handschriften der antiken Aerzte" of the Prussian Academy, edited by Diels (Berlin, 1905). The Prussian Academy has undertaken the editorship of the "Corpus Medicorum Graecorum." There is no complete edition of them in English. In 1849 the Deeside physician, Adams, published (for the Old Sydenham Society) a translation of the most important works, a valuable edition and easily obtained. Littre's ten-volume edition "OEuvres completes d'Hippocrate," Paris, 1839-1861, is the most important for reference. Those of you who want a brief but very satisfactory account of the Hippocratic writings, with numerous extracts, will find the volume of Theodor Beck (Jena, 1907) very useful.

I can only indicate, in a very brief way, the special features of the Hippocratic writings that have influenced the evolution of the science and art of medicine.

The first is undoubtedly the note of humanity. In his introduction to, "The Rise of the Greek Epic,"(21) Gilbert Murray emphasizes the idea of service to the community as more deeply rooted in the Greeks than in us. The question they asked about each writer was, "Does he help to make better men?" or "Does he make life a better thing?" Their aim was to be useful, to be helpful, to make better men in the cities, to correct life, "to make gentle the life of the world." In this brief phrase were summed up the aspirations of the Athenians, likewise illuminated in that remarkable saying of Prodicus (fifth century B.C.), "That which benefits human life is God." The

Greek view of man was the very antithesis of that which St. Paul enforced upon the Christian world. One idea pervades thought from Homer to Lucian-like an aroma—pride in the body as a whole. In the strong conviction that "our soul in its rose mesh" is quite as much helped by flesh as flesh by the soul the Greek sang his song—"For pleasant is this flesh." Just so far as we appreciate the value of the fair mind in the fair body, so far do we apprehend ideals expressed by the Greek in every department of life. The beautiful soul harmonizing with the beautiful body was as much the glorious ideal of Plato as it was the end of the education of Aristotle. What a splendid picture in Book III of the "Republic," of the day when ". . . our youth will dwell in a land of health, amid fair sights and sounds and receive the good in everything; and beauty, the effluence of fair works, shall flow into the eye and ear like a health-giving breeze from a purer region, and insensibly draw the soul from earliest years into likeness and sympathy with the beauty of reason." The glory of this zeal for the enrichment of this present life was revealed to the Greeks as to no other people, but in respect to care for the body of the common man, we have only seen its fulfilment in our own day, as a direct result of the methods of research initiated by them. Everywhere throughout the Hippocratic writings we find this attitude towards life, which has never been better expressed than in the fine phrase, "Where there is love of humanity there will be love of the profession." This is well brought out in the qualifications laid down by Hippocrates for the study of medicine. "Whoever is to acquire a competent knowledge of medicine ought to be possessed of the following advantages: a natural disposition; instruction; a favourable position for the study; early tuition; love of labour; leisure. First of all, a natural talent is required, for when nature opposes, everything else is vain; but when nature leads the way to what is most excellent, instruction in the art takes place, which the student must try to appropriate to himself by reflection, becoming a nearly pupil in a place well adapted for instruction. He must also bring to the task a love of labour and perseverance, so that the instruction taking root may bring forth proper and abundant fruits." And the directions given for the conduct of life and for the relation which the physician should have with the public are those of our code of ethics today. Consultations in doubtful cases are advised, touting for fees is discouraged. "If two or more ways of medical treatment were possible, the physician was recommended to choose the least imposing or sensational; it was an act of 'deceit' to dazzle the patient's eye by brilliant exhibitions of skill which might very well be dispensed with. The practice of holding public lectures in order to increase his reputation was discouraged in the physician, and he was especially warned against lectures tricked out with quotations from the poets. Physicians who pretended to infallibility in detecting even the minutest departure from their prescriptions were laughed at; and finally, there were precise by-laws to regulate the personal behaviour of the physician. He was enjoined to observe the most scrupulous cleanliness, and was advised to cultivate an elegance removed from all signs of luxury, even down to the detail that he might use perfumes, but not in an immoderate degree "(22) But the high-water mark of professional morality is reached in the famous Hippocratic oath, which Gomperz calls "a monument of the highest rank in the history of civilization." It is of small matter whether this is of Hippocratic date or not, or whether it has in it Egyptian or Indian elements: its importance lies in the accuracy with which it represents the Greek spirit. For twenty-five centuries it has been the "credo" of the profession, and in many universities it is still the formula with which men are admitted to the doctorate.

(21) Oxford. Clarendon Press, 2d ed., 1911.

(22) Gomperz Greek Thinkers, Vol. I, p. 281.

I swear by Apollo the physician and AEsculapius and Health (Hygieia) and Al-Heal (Panacea) and all the gods and goddesses, that, according to my ability and judgment, I will keep this oath and this stipulation—to reckon him who taught me this art equally dear to me as my parents, to share my substance with him, and relieve his necessities if required; to look upon his offspring in the same footing as my own brothers, and to teach them this art, if they shall wish to learn it, without fee or stipulation; and that by precept, lecture, and every other mode of instruction, I will impart a knowledge of my art to my own sons, and those of my teachers, and to disciples bound by a stipulation and oath according to the law of medicine, but to none others. I will follow that system of regimen which, according to my ability and judgement, I consider for the benefit of my patients, and abstain from whatever is deleterious and mischievous.

I will give no deadly medicine to anyone if asked, nor suggest any such counsel; and in like manner I will not give to a woman a pessary to produce abortion.

With purity and with holiness I will pass my life and practice my art.

(I will not cut persons labouring under the stone, but will leave this to be done by men who are practitioners of this work.)

Into whatsoever houses I enter, I will go into them for the benefit of the sick and will abstain from every voluntary act of mischief and corruption, and, further, from the abduction of females or males, of freemen and slaves. Whatever, in connection with my professional practice, or not in connection with it, I see or hear, in the life of men, which ought not to be spoken of abroad, I will not divulge, as reckoning that all such should be kept secret.

While I continue to keep this Oath unviolated, may it be granted to me to enjoy life and the practice of the art, respected by all men, in all times! But should I trespass and violate this Oath, may the reverse be my lot!

(Adams, II, 779, cf. Littre, IV, 628.)

In his ideal republic, Plato put the

physician low enough, in the last stratum, indeed, but he has never been more honorably placed than in the picture of Athenian society given by this author in the "Symposium." Here the physician is shown as a cultivated gentleman, mixing in the best, if not always the most sober, society. Eryximachus, the son of Acumenus, himself a physician, plays in this famous scene a typical Greek part(22a)—a strong advocate of temperance in mind and body, deprecating, as a physician, excess in drink, he urged that conversation should be the order of the day and he had the honor of naming the subject—"Praise of the God of Love." Incidentally Eryximachus gives his view of the nature of disease, and shows how deeply he was influenced by the views of Empedocles:". . . so too in the body the good and healthy elements are to be indulged, and the bad elements and the elements of disease are not to be indulged, but discouraged. And this is what the physician has to do, and in this the art of medicine consists: for medicine may be regarded generally as the knowledge of the loves and desires of the body and how to satisfy them or not; and the best physician is he who is able to separate fair love from foul, or to convert one into the other; and he who knows how to eradicate and how to implant love, whichever is required, and can reconcile the most hostile elements in the constitution and make them loving friends, is a skilful practitioner."

(22a) Professor Gildersleeve's view of Eryximachus is less
    favorable (Johns Hopkins University Circular, Baltimore,
    January, 1887). Plato, III, 186— Jowett, I, 556.

The second great note in Greek medicine illustrates the directness with which they went to the very heart of the matter. Out of mysticism, superstition and religious ritual the Greek went directly to nature and was the first to grasp the conception of medicine as an art based on accurate observation, and an integral part of the science of man. What could be more striking than the phrase in "The Law," "There are, in effect, two things, to know and to believe one knows; to know is science; to believe one knows is ignorance"?(23) But no single phrase in the writings can compare for directness with the famous aphorism which has gone into the literature of all lands: "Life is short and Art is long; the Occasion fleeting, Experience fallacious, and Judgment difficult."

(23) Littre: OEuvres d'Hippocrate, Vol. IV, pp. 641-642.

Everywhere one finds a strong, clear common sense, which refuses to be entangled either in theological or philosophical speculations. What Socrates did for philosophy Hippocrates may be said to have done for medicine. As Socrates devoted himself to ethics, and the application of right thinking to good conduct, so Hippocrates insisted upon the practical nature of the art, and in placing its highest good in the benefit of the patient. Empiricism, experience, the collection of facts, the evidence of the senses, the avoidance of philosophical speculations, were the distinguishing features of Hippocratic medicine. One of the most striking contributions of Hippocrates is the recognition that diseases are only part of the processes of nature, that there is nothing divine or sacred about them. With reference to epilepsy, which was regarded as a sacred disease, he says, "It appears to me to be no wise more divine nor more sacred than other diseases, but has a natural cause from which it originates like other affections; men regard its nature and cause as divine from ignorance." And in another place he remarks that each disease has its own nature, and that no one arises without a natural cause. He seems to have been the first to grasp the conception of the great healing powers of nature. In his long experience with the cures in the temples, he must have seen scores of instances in which the god had worked the miracle through the vis medicatrix naturae; and to the shrewd wisdom of his practical suggestions in treatment may be attributed in large part the extraordinary vogue which the great Coan has enjoyed for twenty-five centuries. One may appreciate the veneration with which the Father of Medicine was regarded by the attribute "divine" which was usually attached to his name. Listen to this for directness and honesty of speech taken from the work on the joints characterized by Littre as "the great surgical monument of antiquity": "I have written this down deliberately, believing it is valuable to learn of unsuccessful experiments, and to know the causes of their non-success."

The note of freedom is not less remarkable throughout the Hippocratic writings, and it is not easy to understand how a man brought up and practicing within the precincts of a famous AEsculapian temple could have divorced himself so wholly from the superstitions and vagaries of the cult. There are probably grounds for Pliny's suggestion that he benefited by the receipts written in the temple, registered by the sick cured of any disease. "Afterwards," Pliny goes on to remark in his characteristic way, "hee professed that course of Physicke which is called Clinice Wherby physicians found such sweetnesse that afterwards there was no measure nor end of fees," ('Natural History,' XXIX, 1). There is no reference in the Hippocratic writings to divination; incubation sleep is not often mentioned, and charms, incantations or the practice of astrology but rarely. Here and there we do find practices which jar upon modern feeling, but on the whole we feel in reading the Hippocratic writings nearer to their spirit than to that of the Arabians or of the many writers of the fifteenth and sixteenth centuries A. D. And it is not only against the thaumaturgic powers that the Hippocratic writings protested, but they express an equally active reaction against the excesses and defects of the new philosophy, a point brought out very clearly by Gomperz.(24) He regards it as an undying glory of the school of Cos that after years of vague, restless speculation it introduces "steady sedentary habits into the intellectual life of mankind." 'Fiction to the right! Reality to the left!' was the battlecry of this school in the war they were the first to wage against the excesses and defects of the nature-philosophy. Though the protest was effective in certain directions, we shall see that the authors of the Hippocratic writings could not entirely escape from the hypotheses of the older philosophers.

(24) Gomperz Greek Thinkers, Vol. I, p. 296.

I can do no more than indicate in the briefest possible way some of the more important views ascribed to Hippocrates. We cannot touch upon the disputes between the Coan and Cnidian schools.(25) You must bear in mind that the Greeks at this time had no human anatomy. Dissections were impossible; their physiology was of the crudest character, strongly dominated by the philosophies. Empedocles regarded the four elements, fire, air, earth and water, as "the roots of all things," and this became the corner stone in the humoral pathology of Hippocrates. As in the Macrocosm—the world at large there were four elements, fire, air, earth, and water, so in the Microcosm—the world of man's body—there were four humors (elements), viz., blood, phlegm, yellow bile (or choler) and black bile (or melancholy), and they corresponded to the four qualities of matter, heat, cold, dryness and moisture. For more than two thousand years these views prevailed. In his "Regiment of Life" (1546) Thomas Phaer says:". . . which humours are called ye sones of the Elements because they be complexioned like the foure Elements, for like as the Ayre is hot and moyst: so is the blooud, hote and moyste. And as Fyer is hote and dry: so is Cholere hote and dry. And as water is colde and moyst: so is fleume colde and moyste. And as the Earth is colde and dry: so Melancholy is colde and dry."(26)

(25) The student who wishes a fuller account is referred to
  the histories of (a) Neuburger, Vol. 1, Oxford, 1910; (b)
  Withington, London, 1894.

(26) Thomas Phaer: Regiment of Life, London, 1546.

As the famous Regimen Sanitatis of Salernum, the popular family handbook of the Middle Ages, says:

Foure Humours raigne within our bodies wholly,
And these compared to foure elements.(27)

(27) The Englishman's Doctor, or the Schoole of Salerne, Sir
  John Harington's translation, London, 1608, p. 2. Edited by
  Francis R. Packard, New York, 1920, p. 132. Harington's book
  originally appeared dated: London 1607. (Hoe copy in the
  Henry E. Huntington Library.)

According to Littre, there is nowhere so strong a statement of these views in the genuine works of Hippocrates, but they are found at large in the Hippocratic writings, and nothing can be clearer than the following statement from the work "The Nature of Man": "The body of man contains in itself blood and phlegm and yellow bile and black bile, which things are in the natural constitution of his body, and the cause of sickness and of health. He is healthy when they are in proper proportion between one another as regards mixture and force and quantity, and when they are well mingled together; he becomes sick when one of these is diminished or increased in amount, or is separated in the body from its proper mixture, and not properly mingled with all the others." No words could more clearly express the views of disease which, as I mentioned, prevailed until quite recent years. The black bile, melancholy, has given us a great word in the language, and that we have not yet escaped from the humoral pathology of Hippocrates is witnessed by the common expression of biliousness—"too much bile"—or "he has a touch of the liver." The humors, imperfectly mingled, prove irritant in the body. They are kept in due proportion by the innate heat which, by a sort of internal coction gradually changes the humors to their proper proportion. Whatever may be the primary cause of the change in the humors manifesting itself in disease, the innate heat, or as Hippocrates terms it, the nature of the body itself, tends to restore conditions to the norm; and this change occurring suddenly, or abruptly, he calls the "crisis," which is accomplished on some special day of the disease, and is often accompanied by a critical discharge, or by a drop in the body temperature. The evil, or superabundant, humors were discharged and this view of a special materies morbi, to be got rid of by a natural processor a crisis, dominated pathology until quite recently. Hippocrates had a great belief in the power of nature, the vis medicatrix naturae, to restore the normal state. A keen observer and an active practitioner, his views of disease, thus hastily sketched, dominated the profession for twenty-five centuries; indeed, echoes of his theories are still heard in the schools, and his very words are daily on our lips. If asked what was the great contribution to medicine of Hippocrates and his school we could answer—the art of careful observation.

In the Hippocratic writings is summed up the experience of Greece to the Golden Age of Pericles. Out of philosophy, out of abstract speculation, had come a way of looking at nature for which the physicians were mainly responsible, and which has changed forever men's views on disease. Medicine broke its leading strings to religion and philosophy—a tottering, though lusty, child whose fortunes we are to follow in these lectures. I have a feeling that, could we know more of the medical history of the older races of which I spoke in the first lecture, we might find that this was not the first-born of Asklepios, that there had been many premature births, many still-born offspring, even live-births—the products of the fertilization of nature by the human mind, but the record is dark, and the infant was cast out like Israel in the chapter of Isaiah. But the high-water mark of mental achievement had not been reached by the great generation in which Hippocrates had labored. Socrates had been dead sixteen years, and Plato was a man of forty-five, when far away in the north in the little town of Stagira, on the peninsula of Mount Athos in Macedoniawas, in 384 B.C., born a "man of men," the one above all others to whom the phrase of Milton may be applied. The child of an Asklepiad, Nicomachus, physician to the father of Philip, there must have been a rare conjunction of the planets at the birth of the great Stagirite. In the first circle of the "Inferno," Virgil leads Dante into a wonderful company, "star-seated" on the verdure (he says)—the philosophic family looking with reverence on "the Master of those who know"—il maestro di color che sanno.(28) And with justice has Aristotle been so regarded for these twenty-three centuries. No man has ever swayed such an intellectual empire—in logic, metaphysics, rhetoric, psychology, ethics, poetry, politics and natural history, in all a creator, and in all still a master. The history of the human mind—offers no parallel to his career. As the creator of the sciences of comparative anatomy, systematic zoology, embryology, teratology, botany and physiology, his writings have an eternal interest. They present an extraordinary accumulation of facts relating to the structure and functions of various parts of the body. It is an unceasing wonder how one man, even with a school of devoted students, could have done so much.

(28) The "Good collector of qualities," Dioscorides,
  Hippocrates, Avicenna, Galen and Averroes were the medical
  members of the group. Dante, Inferno, canto iv.

Dissection—already practiced by Alcmaeon, Democritus, Diogenes and others—was conducted on a large scale, but the human body was still taboo. Aristotle confesses that the "inward parts of man are known least of all," and he had never seen the human kidneys or uterus. In his physiology, I can refer to but one point—the pivotal question of the heart and blood vessels. To Aristotle the heart was the central organ controlling the circulation, the seat of vitality, the source of the blood, the place in which it received its final elaboration and impregnation with animal heat. The blood was contained in the heart and vessels as in a vase—hence the use of the term "vessel." "From the heart the blood-vessels extend throughout the body as in the anatomical diagrams which are represented on the walls, for the parts lie round these because they are formed out of them."(29) The nutriment oozes through the blood vessels and the passages in each of the parts "like water in unbaked pottery." He did not recognize any distinction between arteries and veins, calling both plebes (Littre); the vena cava is the great vessel, and the aorta the smaller; but both contain blood. He did not use the word "arteria" (arthria) for either of them. There was no movement from the heart to the vessels but the blood was incessantly drawn upon by the substance of the body and as unceasingly renewed by absorption of the products of digestion, the mesenteric vessels taking up nutriment very much as the plants take theirs by the roots from the soil. From the lungs was absorbed the pneuma, or spiritus, which was conveyed to the heart by the pulmonary vessels—one to the right, and one to the left side. These vessels in the lungs, "through mutual contact" with the branches of the trachea, took in the pneuma. A point of interest is that the windpipe, or trachea, is called "arteria," both by Aristotle and by Hippocrates ("Anatomy," Littre, VII, 539). It was the air-tube, disseminating the breath through the lungs. We shall see in a few minutes how the term came to be applied to the arteries, as we know them. The pulsation of the heart and arteries was regarded by Aristotle as a sort of ebullition in which the liquids were inflated by the vital or innate heat, the fires of which were cooled by the pneuma taken in by the lungs and carried to the heart by the pulmonary vessels.

(29) De Generatione Animalium, Oxford translation, Bk. II,
  Chap. 6, Works V, 743 a.

In Vol. IV of Gomperz' "Greek Thinkers," you will find an admirable discussion on Aristotle as an investigator of nature, and those of you who wish to study his natural history works more closely may do so easily—in the new translation which is in process of publication by the Clarendon Press, Oxford. At the end of the chapter "De Respiratione" in the "Parva Naturalia" (Oxford edition, 1908), we have Aristotle's attitude towards medicine expressed in a way worthy of a son of the profession:

"But health and disease also claim the attention of the scientist, and not merely of the physician, in so far as an account of their causes is concerned. The extent to which these two differ and investigate diverse provinces must not escape us, since facts show that their inquiries are, at least to a certain extent, conterminous. For physicians of culture and refinement make some mention of natural science, and claim to derive their principles from it, while the most accomplished investigators into nature generally push their studies so far as to conclude with an account of medical principles." (Works, III, 480 b.)

Theophrastus, a student of Aristotle and his successor, created the science of botany and made possible the pharmacologists of a few centuries later. Some of you doubtless know him in another guise—as the author of the golden booklet on "Characters," in which "the most eminent botanist of antiquity observes the doings of men with the keen and unerring vision of a natural historian" (Gomperz). In the Hippocratic writings, there are mentioned 236 plants; in the botany of Theophrastus, 455. To one trait of master and pupil I must refer—the human feeling, not alone of man for man, but a sympathy that even claims kinship with the animal world. "The spirit with which he (Theophrastus) regarded the animal world found no second expression till the present age" (Gomperz). Halliday, however, makes the statement that Porphyry(30) goes as far as any modern humanitarian in preaching our duty towards animals.

(30) W. R. Halliday: Greek Divination, London, Macmillan &
  Co., 1913.

ALEXANDRIAN SCHOOL

FROM the death of Hippocrates about the year 375 B.C. till the founding of the Alexandrian School, the physicians were engrossed largely in speculative views, and not much real progress was made, except in the matter of elaborating the humoral pathology. Only three or four men of the first rank stand out in this period: Diocles the Carystian, "both in time and reputation next and second to Hippocrates" (Pliny), a keen anatomist and an encyclopaedic writer; but only scanty fragments of his work remain. In some ways the most important member of this group was Praxagoras, a native of Cos, about 340 B.C. Aristotle, you remember, made no essential distinction between arteries and veins, both of which he held to contain blood: Praxagoras recognized that the pulsation was only in the arteries, and maintained that only the veins contained blood, and the arteries air. As a rule the arteries are empty after death, and Praxagoras believed that they were filled with an aeriform fluid, a sort of pneuma, which was responsible for their pulsation. The word arteria, which had already been applied to the trachea, as an air-containing tube, was then attached to the arteries; on account of the rough and uneven character of its walls the trachea was then called the arteria tracheia, or the rough air-tube.(31a) We call it simply the trachea, but in French the word trachee-artere is still used.

(31a) Galen: De usu partium, VII, Chaps. 8-9.

Praxagoras was one of the first to make an exhaustive study of the pulse, and he must have been a man of considerable clinical acumen, as well as boldness, to recommend in obstruction of the bowels the opening of the abdomen, removal of the obstructed portion and uniting the ends of the intestine by sutures.

After the death of Alexander, Egypt fell into the hands of his famous general, Ptolemy, under whose care the city became one of the most important on the Mediterranean. He founded and maintained a museum, an establishment that corresponded very much to a modern university, for the study of literature, science and the arts. Under his successors, particularly the third Ptolemy, the museum developed, more especially the library, which contained more than half a million volumes. The teachers were drawn from all centres, and the names of the great Alexandrians are among the most famous in the history of human knowledge, including such men as Archimedes, Euclid, Strabo and Ptolemy.

In mechanics and physics, astronomy, mathematics and optics, the work of the Alexandrians constitutes the basis of a large part of our modern knowledge. The school-boy of today—or at any rate of my day—studies the identical problems that were set by Euclid 300 B.C., and the student of physics still turns to Archimedes and Heron, and the astronomer to Eratosthenes and Hipparchus. To those of you who wish to get a brief review of the state of science in the Alexandrian School I would recommend the chapter in Vol. I of Dannemann's history.(31)

(31) Friedrich Dannemann:
Grundriss einer Geschichte der
Naturwissenschaften, Vol. I, 3d ed.,
Leipzig, 1908.

Of special interest to us in Alexandria is the growth of the first great medical school of antiquity. Could we have visited the famous museum about 300 B. C., we should have found a medical school in full operation, with extensive laboratories, libraries and clinics. Here for the first time the study of the structure of the human body reached its full development, till then barred everywhere by religious prejudice; but full permission was given by the Ptolemies to perform human dissection and, if we may credit some authors, even vivisection. The original writings of the chief men of this school have not been preserved, but there is a possibility that any day a papyrus maybe found which will supplement the scrappy and imperfect knowledge afforded us by Pliny, Celsus and Galen. The two most distinguished names are Herophilus—who, Pliny says, has the honor of being the first physician "who searched into the causes of disease"—and Erasistratus.

Herophilus, ille anatomicorum coryphaeus, as Vesalius calls him, was a pupil of Praxagoras, and his name is still in everyday use by medical students, attached to the torcular Herophili. Anatomy practically dates from these Alexandrines, who described the valves of the heart, the duodenum, and many of the important parts of the brain; they recognized the true significance of the nerves (which before their day had been confounded with the tendons), distinguished between motor and sensory nerves, and regarded the brain as the seat of the perceptive faculties and voluntary action. Herophilus counted the pulse, using the water-clock for the purpose, and made many subtle analyses of its rate and rhythm; and, influenced by the musical theories of the period, he built up a rhythmical pulse lore which continued in medicine until recent times. He was a skilful practitioner and to him is ascribed the statement that drugs are the hands of the gods. There is a very modern flavor to his oft-quoted expression that the best physician was the man who was able to distinguish between the possible and the impossible.

Erasistratus elaborated the view of the pneuma, one form of which he believed came from the inspired air, and passed to the left side of the heart and to the arteries of the body. It was the cause of the heart-beat and the source of the innate heat of the body, and it maintained the processes of digestion and nutrition. This was the vital spirit; the animal spirit was elaborated in the brain, chiefly in the ventricles, and sent by the nerves to all parts of the body, endowing the individual with life and perception and motion. In this way a great division was made between the two functions of the body, and two sets of organs: in the vascular system, the heart and arteries and abdominal organs, life was controlled by the vital spirits; on the other hand, in the nervous system were elaborated the animal spirits, controlling motion, sensation and the various special senses. These views on the vital and animal spirits held unquestioned sway until well into the eighteenth century, and we still, in a measure, express the views of the great Alexandrian when we speak of "high" or "low" spirits.

GALEN

PERGAMON has become little more than a name associated in our memory with the fulminations of St. John against the seven churches of Asia; and on hearing the chapter read, we wondered what was "Satan's seat" and who were the "Nicolaitanes" whose doctrine he so hated. Renewed interest has been aroused in the story of its growth and of its intellectual rivalry with Alexandria since the wonderful discoveries by German archaeologists which have enabled us actually to see this great Ionian capital, and even the "seat of Satan." The illustration here shown is of the famous city, in which you can see the Temple of Athena Polis on the rock, and the amphitheatre. Its interest for us is connected with the greatest name, after Hippocrates, in Greek medicine, that of Galen, born at Pergamon A. D. 130, in whom was united as never before—and indeed one may say, never since—the treble combination of observer, experimenter and philosopher. His father, Nikon, a prosperous architect, was urged in a dream to devote his son to the profession of medicine, upon which study the lad entered in his seventeenth year under Satyrus. In his writings, Galen gives many details of his life, mentioning the names of his teachers, and many incidents in his Wanderjahre, during which he studied at the best medical schools, including Alexandria. Returning to his native city he was put in charge of the gladiators, whose wounds he said he treated with wine. In the year 162, he paid his first visit to Rome, the scene of his greatest labors. Here he gave public lectures on anatomy, and became "the fashion." He mentions many of his successes; one of them is the well-worn story told also of Erasistratus and Stratonice, but Galen's story is worth telling, and it is figured as a miniature in the manuscripts of his works. Called to see a lady he found her suffering from general malaise without any fever or increased action of the pulse. He saw at once that her trouble was mental and, like a wise physician, engaged her in general conversation. Quite possibly he knew her story, for the name of a certain actor, Pylades, was mentioned, and he noticed that her pulse at once increased in rapidity and became irregular. On the next day he arranged that the name of another actor, Morphus, should be mentioned, and on the third day the experiment was repeated but without effect. Then on the fourth evening it was again mentioned that Pylades was dancing, and the pulse quickened and became irregular, so he concluded that she was in love with Pylades. He tells how he was first called to treat the Emperor Marcus Aurelius, who had a stomach-ache after eating too much cheese. He treated the case so successfully that the Emperor remarked, "I have but one physician, and he is a gentleman." He seems to have had good fees, as he received 400 aurei (about 2000) for a fortnight's attendance upon the wife of Boethus.

He left Rome for a time in 168 A. D. and returned to Pergamon, but was recalled to Rome by the Emperor, whom he accompanied on an expedition to Germany. There are records in his writings of many journeys, and busy with his practice in dissections and experiments he passed a long and energetic life, dying, according to most authorities, in the year 200 A.D.

A sketch of the state of medicine in Rome is given by Celsus in the first of his eight books, and he mentions the names of many of the leading practitioners, particularly Asclepiades, the Bithynian, a man of great ability, and a follower of the Alexandrians, who regarded all disease as due to a disturbed movement of the atoms. Diet, exercise, massage and bathing were his great remedies, and his motto—tuto, cito et jucunde—has been the emulation of all physicians. How important a role he and his successors played until the time of Galen may be gathered from the learned lectures of Sir Clifford Allbutt(32) on "Greek Medicine in Rome" and from Meyer-Steineg's "Theodorus Priscianus und die romische Medizin."(33) From certain lay writers we learn that it was the custom for popular physicians to be followed on their rounds by crowds of students. Martial's epigram (V, ix) is often referred to:

Languebam: sed tu comitatus protinus ad me
  Venisti centum, Symmache, discipulis.
  Centum me tegigere manus Aquilone gelatae
  Non habui febrem, Symmache, nunc habeo.

(32) Allbutt: British Medical Journal, London, 1909, ii, 1449; 1515; 1598.

(33) Fischer, Jena, 1909.

And in the "Apollonius of Tyana" by Philostratus, when Apollonius wishes to prove an alibi, he calls to witness the physicians of his sick friend, Seleucus and Straloctes, who were accompanied by their clinical class to the number of about thirty students.(34) But for a first-hand sketch of the condition of the profession we must go to Pliny, whose account in the twenty-ninth book of the "Natural History" is one of the most interesting and amusing chapters in that delightful work. He quotes Cato's tirade against Greek physicians,—corrupters of the race, whom he would have banished from the city,—then he sketches the career of some of the more famous of the physicians under the Empire, some of whom must have had incomes never approached at any other period in the history of medicine. The chapter gives a good picture of the stage on which Galen (practically a contemporary of Pliny) was to play so important a role. Pliny seems himself to have been rather disgusted with the devious paths of the doctors of his day, and there is no one who has touched with stronger language upon the weak points of the art of physic. In one place he says that it alone has this peculiar art and privilege, "That whosoever professeth himself a physician, is straightwaies beleeved, say what he will: and yet to speake a truth, there are no lies dearer sold or more daungerous than those which proceed out of a Physician's mouth. Howbeit, we never once regard or look to that, so blind we are in our deepe persuasion of them, and feed our selves each one in a sweet hope and plausible conceit of our health by them. Moreover, this mischief there is besides, That there is no law or statute to punish the ignorance of blind Physicians, though a man lost his life by them: neither was there ever any man knowne, who had revenge of recompence for the evil intreating or misusage under their hands. They learne their skill by endaungering our lives: and to make proofe and experiments of their medicines, they care not to kill us. "(35) He says it is hard that, while the judges are carefully chosen and selected, physicians are practically their own judges, and that of the men who may give us a quick despatch and send us to Heaven or Hell, no enquiry or examination is made of their quality and worthiness. It is interesting to read so early a bitter criticism of the famous "Theriaca," a great compound medicine invented by Antiochus III, which had a vogue for fifteen hundred years.

(34) Bk. VIII, Chap. VII.

(35) Pliny: Natural History (XXIX, 1), Philemon Holland's
version, London, 1601, II, 347.

But we must return to Galen and his works, which comprise the most voluminous body of writings left by any of the ancients. The great edition is that in twenty-two volumes by Kuhn (1821-1833). The most useful editions are the "Juntines" of Venice, which were issued in thirteen editions. In the fourth and subsequent editions a very useful index by Brassavola is included. A critical study of the writings is at present being made by German scholars for the Prussian Academy, which will issue a definitive edition of his works.

Galen had an eclectic mind and could not identify himself with any of the prevailing schools, but regarded himself as a disciple of Hippocrates. For our purpose, both his philosophy and his practice are of minor interest in comparison with his great labors in anatomy and physiology.

In anatomy, he was a pupil of the Alexandrians to whom he constantly refers. Times must have changed since the days of Herophilus, as Galen does not seem ever to have had an opportunity of dissecting the human body, and he laments the prejudice which prevents it. In the study of osteology, he urges the student to be on the lookout for an occasional human bone exposed in a graveyard, and on one occasion he tells of finding the carcass of a robber with the bones picked bare by birds and beasts. Failing this source, he advises the student to go to Alexandria, where there were still two skeletons. He himself dissected chiefly apes and pigs. His osteology was admirable, and his little tractate "De Ossibus" could, with very few changes, be used today by a hygiene class as a manual. His description of the muscles and of the organs is very full, covering, of course, many sins of omission and of commission, but it was the culmination of the study of the subject by Greek physicians.

His work as a physiologist was even more important, for, so far as we know, he was the first to carry out experiments on a large scale. In the first place, he was within an ace of discovering the circulation of the blood. You may remember that through the errors of Praxagoras and Erasistratus, the arteries were believed to contain air and got their name on that account: Galen showed by experiment that the arteries contain blood and not air. He studied particularly the movements of the heart, the action of the valves, and the pulsatile forces in the arteries. Of the two kinds of blood, the one, contained in the venous system, was dark and thick and rich in grosser elements, and served for the general nutrition of the body. This system took its origin, as is clearly shown in the figure, in the liver, the central organ of nutrition and of sanguification. From the portal system were absorbed, through the stomach and intestines, the products of digestion. From the liver extend the venae cavae, one to supply the head and arms, the other the lower extremities: extending from the right heart was a branch, corresponding to the pulmonary artery, the arterial vein which distributed blood to the lungs. This was the closed venous system. The arterial system, shown, as you see, quite separate in Figure 31, was full of a thinner, brighter, warmer blood, characterized by the presence of an abundance of the vital spirits. Warmed in the ventricle, it distributed vital heat to all parts of the body. The two systems were closed and communicated with each other only through certain pores or perforations in the septum separating the ventricles. At the periphery, however, Galen recognized (as had been done already by the Alexandrians) that the arteries anastomose with the veins, ". . . and they mutually receive from each other blood and spirits through certain invisible and extremely small vessels."

It is difficult to understand how Galen missed the circulation of the blood. He knew that the valves of the heart determined the direction of the blood that entered and left the organ, but he did not appreciate that it was a pump for distributing the blood, regarding it rather as a fireplace from which the innate heat of the body was derived. He knew that the pulsatile force was resident in the walls of the heart and in the arteries, and he knew that the expansion, or diastole, drew blood into its cavities, and that the systole forced blood out. Apparently his view was that there was a sort of ebb and flow in both systems—and yet, he uses language just such as we would, speaking of the venous system as ". . . a conduit full of blood with a multitude of canals large and small running out from it and distributing blood to all parts of the body." He compares the mode of nutrition to irrigating canals and gardens, with a wonderful dispensation by nature that they should "neither lack a sufficient quantity of blood for absorption nor be overloaded at any time with excessive supply." The function of respiration was the introduction of the pneuma, the spirits which passed from the lungs to the heart through the pulmonary vessels. Galen went a good deal beyond the idea of Aristotle, reaching our modern conception that the function is to maintain the animal heat, and that the smoky matters derived from combustion of the blood are discharged by expiration.

I have dwelt on these points in Galen's physiology, as they are fundamental in the history of the circulation; and they are sufficient to illustrate his position. Among his other brilliant experiments were the demonstration of the function of the laryngeal nerves, of the motor and sensory functions of the spinal nerve roots, of the effect of transverse incision of the spinal cord, and of the effect of hemisection. Altogether there is no ancient physician in whose writings are contained so many indications of modern methods of research.

Galen's views of disease in general are those of Hippocrates, but he introduces many refinements and subdivisions according to the predominance of the four humors, the harmonious combination of which means health, or eucrasia, while their perversion or improper combination leads to dyscrasia, or ill health. In treatment he had not the simplicity of Hippocrates: he had great faith in drugs and collected plants from all parts of the known world, for the sale of which he is said to have had a shop in the neighborhood of the Forum. As I mentioned, he was an eclectic, held himself aloof from the various schools of the day, calling no man master save Hippocrates. He might be called a rational empiricist. He made war on the theoretical practitioners of the day, particularly the Methodists, who, like some of their modern followers, held that their business was with the disease and not with the conditions out of which it arose.

No other physician has ever occupied the commanding position of "Clarissimus" Galenus. For fifteen centuries he dominated medical thought as powerfully as did Aristotle in the schools. Not until the Renaissance did daring spirits begin to question the infallibility of this medical pope. But here we must part with the last and, in many ways, the greatest of the Greeks—a man very much of our own type, who, could he visit this country today, might teach us many lessons. He would smile in scorn at the water supply of many of our cities, thinking of the magnificent aqueducts of Rome and of many of the colonial towns—some still in use—which in lightness of structure and in durability testify to the astonishing skill of their engineers. There are country districts in which he would find imperfect drainage and could tell of the wonderful system by which Rome was kept sweet and clean. Nothing would delight him more than a visit to Panama to see what the organization of knowledge has been able to accomplish. Everywhere he could tour the country as a sanitary expert, preaching the gospel of good water supply and good drainage, two of the great elements in civilization, in which in many places we have not yet reached the Roman standard.

CHAPTER III — MEDIAEVAL MEDICINE

THERE are waste places of the earth which fill one with terror—not simply because they are waste; one has not such feelings in the desert nor in the vast solitude of the ocean. Very different is it where the desolation has overtaken a brilliant and flourishing product of man's head and hand. To know that

> . . . the Lion and the Lizard keep
> The Courts where Jamshyd gloried and drank deep

sends a chill to the heart, and one trembles with a sense of human instability. With this feeling we enter the Middle Ages. Following the glory that was Greece and the grandeur that was Rome, a desolation came upon the civilized world, in which the light of learning burned low, flickering almost to extinction. How came it possible that the gifts of Athens and of Alexandria were deliberately thrown away? For three causes. The barbarians shattered the Roman Empire to its foundations. When Alaric entered Rome in 410 A. D., ghastly was the impression made on the contemporaries; the Roman world shuddered in a titanic spasm (Lindner). The land was a garden of Eden before them, behind a howling wilderness, as is so graphically told in Gibbon's great history. Many of the most important centres of learning were destroyed, and for centuries Minerva and Apollo forsook the haunts of men. The other equally important cause was the change wrought by Christianity. The brotherhood of man, the care of the body, the gospel of practical virtues formed the essence of the teaching of the Founder—in these the Kingdom of Heaven was to be sought; in these lay salvation. But the world was very evil, all thought that the times were waxing late, and into men's minds entered as never before a conviction of the importance of the four last things—death, judgment, heaven and hell. One obstacle alone stood between man and his redemption, the vile body, "this muddy vesture of decay," that so grossly wrapped his soul. To find methods of bringing it into subjection was the task of the Christian Church for centuries. In the Vatican Gallery of Inscriptions is a stone slab with the single word "Stercoriae," and below, the Christian symbol. It might serve as a motto for the Middle Ages, during which, to quote St. Paul, all things were "counted dung but to win Christ." In this attitude of mind the wisdom of the Greeks was not simply foolishness, but a stumbling-block in the path. Knowledge other than that which made a man "wise unto salvation" was useless. All that was necessary was contained in the Bible or taught by the Church. This simple creed brought consolation to thousands and illumined the lives of some of the noblest of men. But, "in seeking a heavenly home man lost his bearings upon earth." Let me commend for your reading Taylor's "Mediaeval Mind."(1) I cannot judge of its scholarship, which I am told by scholars is ripe and good, but I can judge of its usefulness for anyone who wishes to know the story of the mind of man in Europe at this period. Into the content of mediaeval thought only a mystic can enter with full sympathy. It was a needful change in the evolution of the race. Christianity brought new ideals and new motives into the lives of men. The world's desire was changed, a desire for the Kingdom of Heaven, in the search for which the lust of the flesh, the lust of the eye and the pride of life were as dross. A master-motive swayed the minds of sinful men and a zeal to save other souls occupied the moments not devoted to the perfection of their own. The new dispensation made any other superfluous. As Tertullian said: Investigation since the Gospel is no longer necessary. (Dannemann, Die Naturw., I, p. 214) The attitude of the early Fathers toward the body is well expressed by Jerome. "Does your skin roughen without baths? Who is once washed in the blood of Christ needs not wash again." In this unfavorable medium for its growth, science was simply disregarded, not in any hostile spirit, but as unnecessary.(2) And a third contributing factor was the plague of the sixth century, which desolated the whole Roman world. On the top of the grand mausoleum of Hadrian, visitors at Rome see the figure of a gilded angel with a drawn sword, from which the present name of the Castle of St. Angelo takes its origin. On the twenty-fifth of April, 590, there set out from the Church of SS. Cosmas and Damian, already the Roman patron saints of medicine, a vast procession, led by St. Gregory the Great, chanting a seven-fold litany of intercession against the plague. The legend relates that Gregory saw on the top of Hadrian's tomb an angel with a drawn sword, which he sheathed as the plague abated.

(1) H. O. Taylor: The Mediaeval Mind, 2 vols., Macmillan Co.,
New York, 1911. (New edition, 1920.)

(2) Ibid., Vol. 1, p. 13: "Under their action (the Christian
Fathers) the peoples of Western Europe, from the eighth to the
thirteenth century, passed through a homogeneous growth, and
evolved a spirit different from that of any other period of
history—a spirit which stood in awe before its monitors divine
and human, and deemed that knowledge was to be drawn from the
storehouse of the past; which seemed to rely on everything except
its sin-crushed self, and trusted everything except its senses;
which in the actual looked for the ideal, in the concrete saw the
symbol, in the earthly Church beheld the heavenly, and in fleshly
joys discerned the devil's lures; which lived in the unreconciled
opposition between the lust and vain-glory of earth and the
attainment of salvation; which felt life's terror and its
pitifulness, and its eternal hope; around which waved concrete
infinitudes, and over which flamed the terror of darkness and the
Judgment Day."

Galen died about 200 A.D.; the high-water mark of the Renaissance, so far as medicine is concerned, was reached in the year 1542. In order to traverse this long interval intelligently, I will sketch certain great movements, tracing the currents of Greek thought, setting forth in their works the lives of certain great leaders, until we greet the dawn of our own day.

After flowing for more than a thousand years through the broad plain of Greek civilization, the stream of scientific medicine which we have been following is apparently lost in the morass of the Middle Ages; but, checked and blocked like the White Nile in the Soudan, three channels may be followed through the weeds of theological and philosophical speculation.

SOUTH ITALIAN SCHOOL

A WIDE stream is in Italy, where the "antique education never stopped, antique reminiscence and tradition never passed away, and the literary matter of the pagan past never faded from the consciousness of the more educated among the laity and clergy."(3) Greek was the language of South Italy and was spoken in some of its eastern towns until the thirteenth century. The cathedral and monastic schools served to keep alive the ancient learning. Monte Casino stands pre-eminent as a great hive of students, and to the famous Regula of St. Benedict(4) we are indebted for the preservation of many precious manuscripts.

(3) H. O. Taylor: The Mediaeval Mind, Vol. I, p. 251.

(4) De Renzi: Storia Documentata della Scuola Medica di Salerno,
2d ed., Napoli, 1867, Chap. V.

The Norman Kingdom of South Italy and Sicily was a meeting ground of Saracens, Greeks and Lombards. Greek, Arabic and Latin were in constant use among the people of the capital, and Sicilian scholars of the twelfth century translated directly from the Greek.

The famous "Almagest" of Ptolemy, the most important work of ancient astronomy, was translated from a Greek manuscript, as early as 1160, by a medical student of Salerno.(5)

(5) Haskins and Lockwood: Harvard Studies in Classical
Philology, 1910, XXI, pp. 75-102.

About thirty miles southeast of Naples lay Salernum, which for centuries kept alight the lamp of the old learning, and became the centre of medical studies in the Middle Ages; well deserving its name of "Civitas Hippocratica." The date of foundation is uncertain, but Salernitan physicians are mentioned as early as the middle of the ninth century, and from this date until the rise of the universities it was not only a great medical school, but a popular resort for the sick and wounded. As the scholar says in Longfellow's "Golden Legend":

Then at every season of the year
There are crowds of guests and

travellers here;
   Pilgrims and mendicant friars and traders
   From the Levant, with figs and wine,
   And bands of wounded and sick Crusaders,
   Coming back from Palestine.

There were medical and surgical clinics, foundling hospitals, Sisters of Charity, men and women professors—among the latter the famous Trotula—and apothecaries. Dissections were carried out, chiefly upon animals, and human subjects were occasionally used. In the eleventh and twelfth centuries, the school reached its height, and that remarkable genius, Frederick II, laid down regulations for a preliminary study extending over three years, and a course in medicine for five years, including surgery. Fee tables and strict regulations as to practice were made; and it is specifically stated that the masters were to teach in the schools, theoretically and practically, under the authority of Hippocrates and Galen. The literature from the school had a far-reaching influence. One book on the anatomy of the pig illustrates the popular subject for dissection at that time.(6) The writings, which are numerous, have been collected by De Renzi.(7)

(6) "And dissections of the bodies of swine
   As likest the human form divine."—Golden Legend.

(7) S. de Renzi: Collectio Salernitana, 5 vols., Naples,
   1852-1859; P. Giacosa: Magistri Salernitani, Turin, 1901.

The "Antidotarium" of Nicolaus Salernitanus, about 1100, became the popular pharmacopoeia of the Middle Ages, and many modern preparations may be traced to it.

The most prominent man of the school is Constantinus Africanus, a native of Carthage, who, after numerous journeys, reached Salernum about the middle of the eleventh century. He was familiar with the works both of the Greeks and of the Arabs, and it was largely through his translations that the works of Rhazes and Avicenna became known in the West.

One work above all others spread the fame of the school—the Regimen Sanitatis, or Flos Medicinae as it is sometimes called, a poem on popular medicine. It is dedicated to Robert of Normandy, who had been treated at Salernum, and the lines begin: "Anglorum regi scripsit schola tota Salerni . . . " It is a hand-book of diet and household medicine, with many shrewd and taking sayings which have passed into popular use, such as "Joy, temperance and repose Slam the door on the doctor's nose." A full account of the work and the various editions of it is given by Sir Alexander Croke,(8) and the Finlayson lecture (Glasgow Medical Journal, 1908) by Dr. Norman Moore gives an account of its introduction into the British Isles.

(8) Regimen Sanitutis Salernitanum; a Poem on the Preservation of
   Health in Rhyming Latin Verse, Oxford, D.A. Talboys, 1830.

BYZANTINE MEDICINE

THE second great stream which carried Greek medicine to modern days runs through the Eastern Empire. Between the third century and the fall of Constantinople there was a continuous series of Byzantine physicians whose inspiration was largely derived from the old Greek sources. The most distinguished of these was Oribasius, a voluminous compiler, a native of Pergamon and so close a follower of his great townsman that he has been called "Galen's ape." He left many works, an edition of which was edited by Bussemaker and Daremberg. Many facts relating to the older writers are recorded in his writings. He was a contemporary, friend as well as the physician, of the Emperor Julian, for whom he prepared an encyclopaedia of the medical sciences.

Other important Byzantine writers were Aetius and Alexander of Tralles, both of whom were strongly under the influence of Galen and Hippocrates. Their materia medica was based largely upon Dioscorides.

From Byzantium we have the earliest known complete medical manuscript, dating from the fifth century—a work of Dioscorides—one of the most beautiful in existence. It was prepared for Anicia Juliana, daughter of the Emperor of the East, and is now one of the great treasures of the Imperial Library at Vienna.(9) From those early centuries till the fall of Constantinople there is very little of interest medically. A few names stand out prominently, but it is mainly a blank period in our records. Perhaps one man may be mentioned, as he had a great influence on later ages—Actuarius, who lived about 1300, and whose book on the urine laid the foundation of much of the popular uroscopy and water-casting that had such a vogue in the sixteenth and seventeenth centuries. His work on the subject passed through a dozen Latin editions, but is best studied in Ideler's "Physici et medici Graeci minores" (Berlin, 1841).

(9) It has been reproduced by Seatone de Vries, Leyden, 1905,
   Codices graeci et latini photographice depicti, Vol. X.

The Byzantine stream of Greek medicine had dwindled to a very tiny rill when the fall of Constantinople (1453) dispersed to the West many Greek scholars and many precious manuscripts.

ARABIAN MEDICINE

THE third and by far the strongest branch of the Greek river reached the West after a remarkable and meandering course. The map before you shows the distribution of the Graeco-Roman Christian world at the beginning of the seventh century. You will notice that Christianity had extended far eastwards, almost to China. Most of those eastern Christians were Nestorians and one of their important centres was Edessa, whose school of learning became so celebrated. Here in the fifth century was built one of the most celebrated hospitals of antiquity.

Now look at another map showing the same countries about a century later. No such phenomenal change ever was made within so short space of time as that which thus altered the map of Asia and Europe at this period. Within a century, the Crescent had swept from Arabia through the Eastern Empire, over Egypt, North Africa and over Spain in the West, and the fate of Western Europe hung in the balance before the gates of Tours in 732. This time the barbaric horde that laid waste a large part of Christendom were a people that became deeply appreciative of all that was best in Graeco-Roman civilization and of nothing more than of its sciences. The cultivation of medicine was encouraged by the Arabs in a very special way. Anyone wishing to follow the history of the medical profession among this remarkable people will find it admirably presented in Lucien Leclerc's "Histoire de la medecine arabe" (Paris, 1876). An excellent account is also given in Freind's well-known "History of Medicine" (London, 1725-1726). Here I can only indicate very briefly the course of the stream and its freightage.

With the rise of Christianity, Alexandria became a centre of bitter theological and political factions, the story of which haunts the memory of anyone who was so fortunate as to read in his youth Kingsley's "Hypatia." These centuries, with their potent influence of neoplatonism on Christianity, appear to have been sterile enough in medicine. I have already referred to the late Greeks, Aetius and Alexander of Tralles. The last of the Alexandrians was a remarkable man, Paul of AEgina, a great name in medicine and in surgery, who lived in the early part of the seventh century. He also, like Oribasius, was a great compiler. In the year 640, the Arabs took Alexandria, and for the third time a great library was destroyed in the "first city of the West." Shortly after the conquest of Egypt, Greek works were translated into Arabic, often through the medium of Syriac, particularly certain of Galen's books on medicine, and chemical writings, which appear to have laid the foundation of Arabian knowledge on this subject.

Through Alexandria then was one source: but the special development of the Greek science and of medicine took place in the ninth century under the Eastern Caliphates. Let me quote here a couple of sentences from Leclerc (Tome I, pp. 91-92):

"The world has but once witnessed so marvellous a spectacle as that presented by the Arabs in the ninth century. This pastoral people, whose fanaticism had suddenly made them masters of half of the world, having once founded their empire, immediately set themselves to acquire that knowledge of the sciences which alone was lacking to their greatness. Of all the invaders who competed for the last remains of the Roman Empire they alone pursued such studies; while the Germanic hordes, glorying in their brutality and ignorance, took a thousand years to re-unite the broken chain of tradition, the Arabs accomplished this in less than a century. They provoked the competition of the conquered Christians—a healthy competition which secured the harmony of the races.

"At the end of the eighth century, their whole scientific possessions consisted of a translation of one medical treatise and some books on alchemy. Before the ninth century had run to its close, the Arabs were in possession of all the science of the Greeks; they had produced from their own ranks students of the first order, and had raised among their initiators men who, without them, would have been groping in the dark; and they showed from this time an aptitude for the exact sciences, which was lacking in their instructors, whom they henceforward surpassed."

It was chiefly through the Nestorians that the Arabs became acquainted with Greek medicine, and there were two famous families of translators, the Bakhtshuas and the Mesues, both Syrians, and probably not very thoroughly versed in either Greek or Arabic. But the prince of translators, one of the finest figures of the century, was Honein, a Christian Arab, born in 809, whose name was Latinized as Joannitius. "The marvellous extent of his works, their excellence, their importance, the trials he bore nobly at the beginning of his career, everything about him arouses our interest and sympathy. If he did not actually create the Oriental renaissance movement, certainly no one played in it a more active, decided and fruitful part."(10) His industry was colossal. He translated most of the works of Hippocrates and Galen, Aristotle and many others. His famous "Introduction" or "Isagoge," a very popular book in the Middle Ages, is a translation of the "Microtegni" of Galen, a small hand-book, of which a translation is appended to Cholmeley's "John of Gaddesden."(11) The first printed edition of it appeared in 1475 (see Chapter IV at Padua.

(10) Leclerc: Histoire de la medecine arabe, Tome I, p. 139.

(11) Oxford, Clarendon Press, 1912, pp. 136-166. The Mesues also
did great work, and translations of their compilations,
particularly those of the younger Mesue, were widely distributed
in manuscript and were early printed (Venice, 1471) and
frequently reprinted, even as late as the seventeenth century.

Leclerc gives the names of more than one hundred known translators who not only dealt with the physicians but with the Greek philosophers, mathematicians and astronomers. The writings of the physicians of India and of Persia were also translated into Arabic.

But close upon the crowd of translators who introduced the learning of Greece to the Arabians came original observers of the first rank, to a few only of whom time will allow me to refer. Rhazes, so called from the name of the town (Rai) in which he was born, was educated at the great hospital at Bagdad in the second half of the ninth century.

With a true Hippocratic spirit he made many careful observations on disease, and to him we owe the first accurate account of smallpox, which he differentiated from measles. This work was translated for the old Sydenham Society by W.A. Greenhill (1848), and the description given of the disease is well worth reading. He was a man of strong powers of observation, good sense and excellent judgment. His works were very popular, particularly the gigantic "Continens," one of the bulkiest of incunabula. The Brescia edition, 1486, a magnificent volume, extends over 588 pages and it must weigh more than seventeen pounds. It is an encyclopaedia filled with extracts from the Greek and other writers, interspersed with memoranda of his own experiences. His "Almansor" was a very popular text-book, and one of the first to be printed. Book IX of "Almansor" (the name of the prince to whom it was addressed) with the title "De aegritudinibus a capite usque ad pedes," was a very favorite mediaeval text-book. On account of his zeal for study Rhazes was known as the "Experimentator."

The first of the Arabians, known throughout the Middle Ages as the Prince, the rival, indeed, of Galen, was the Persian Ibn Sina, better known as Avicenna, one of the greatest names in the history of medicine. Born about 980 A. D. in the province of Khorasan, near Bokhara, he has left a brief autobiography from which we learn something of his early years. He could repeat the Koran by heart when ten years old, and at twelve he had disputed in law and in logic. So that he found medicine was an easy subject, not hard and thorny like mathematics and metaphysics! He worked night and day, and could solve problems in his dreams. "When I found a difficulty," he says, "I referred to my notes and prayed to the Creator. At night, when weak or sleepy, I strengthened myself with a glass of wine."(12) He was a voluminous writer to whom scores of books are attributed, and he is the author of the most famous medical text-book ever written. It is safe to say that the "Canon" was a medical bible for a longer period than any other work. It "stands for the epitome of all precedent development, the final codification of all Graeco-Arabic medicine. It is a hierarchy of laws liberally illustrated by facts which so ingeniously rule and are subject to one another, stay and uphold one another, that admiration is compelled for the sagacity of the great organiser who, with unparalleled power of systematisation, collecting his material from all sources, constructed so imposing an edifice of fallacy. Avicenna, according to his lights, imparted to contemporary medical science the appearance of almost mathematical accuracy, whilst the art of therapeutics, although empiricism did not wholly lack recognition, was deduced as a logical sequence from theoretical (Galenic and Aristotelian) premises. Is it, therefore, matter for surprise that the majority of investigators and practitioners should have fallen under the spell of this consummation of formalism and should have regarded the 'Canon' as an infallible oracle, the more so in that the logical construction was impeccable and the premises, in the light of contemporary conceptions, passed for incontrovertible axioms?"(13)

(12) Withington: Medical History, London, 1894, pp. 151-152.

(13) Neuburger: History of Medicine, Vol. I, pp. 368-369.

Innumerable manuscripts of it exist: of one of the most beautiful, a Hebrew version (Bologna Library), I give an illustration. A Latin version was printed in 1472 and there are many later editions, the last in 1663. Avicenna was not only a successful writer, but the prototype of the successful physician who was at the same time statesman, teacher, philosopher and literary man. Rumor has it that he became dissipated, and a contemporary saying was that all his philosophy could not make him moral, nor all his physic teach him to preserve his health. He enjoyed a great reputation as a poet. I reproduce a page of a manuscript of one of his poems, which we have in the Bodleian Library. Prof. A.V.W. Jackson says that some of his verse is peculiarly Khayyamesque, though he antedated Omar by a century. That "large Infidel" might well have written such a stanza as

From Earth's dark centre unto Saturn's Gate
I've solved all problems of this world's Estate,
From every snare of Plot and Guile set free,
Each bond resolved, saving alone Death's Fate.

His hymn to the Deity might have been written by Plato and rivals the famous one of Cleanthes.(14) A casual reader gets a very favorable impression of Avicenna. The story of his dominion over the schools in the Middle Ages is one of the most striking in our history. Perhaps we feel that Leclerc exaggerates when he says: "Avicenna is an intellectual phenomenon. Never perhaps has an example been seen of so precocious, quick and wide an intellect extending and asserting itself with so strange and indefatigable an activity." The touch of the man never reached me until I read some of his mystical and philosophical writings translated by Mehren.(15) It is Plato over again. The beautiful allegory in which men are likened to birds snared and caged until set free by the Angel of Death might be met with anywhere in the immortal Dialogues. The tractate on Love is a commentary on the Symposium; and the essay on Destiny is Greek in spirit without a trace of Oriental fatalism, as you may judge from the concluding sentence, which I leave you as his special message: "Take heed to the limits of your capacity and you will arrive at a knowledge of the truth! How true is the saying:—Work ever and to each will come that measure of success for which Nature has designed him." Avicenna died in his fifty-eighth year. When he saw that physic was of no avail, resigning himself to the inevitable, he sold his goods, distributed the money to the poor, read the Koran through once every three days, and died in the holy month of Ramadan. His tomb at Hamadan, the ancient Ecbatana, still exists, a simple brickwork building, rectangular in shape, and surrounded by an unpretentious court. It was restored in 1877, but is again in need of repair. The illustration here shown is from a photograph sent by Dr. Neligan of Teheran. Though dead, the great Persian has still a large practice, as his tomb is much visited by pilgrims, among whom cures are said to be not uncommon.

(14) "L'hymne d'Avicenne" in:
L'Elegie du Tograi, etc., par P.
 Vattier, Paris, 1660.

(15) Traites mystiques d'Abou Ali al-Hosain b. Abdallah b. Sina
ou d'Avicenne par M. A. F.
Mehren, Leyden, E. J. Brill, Fasc.
 I-IV, 1889-1899.

The Western Caliphate produced physicians and philosophers almost as brilliant as those of the East. Remarkable schools of medicine were founded at Seville, Toledo and Cordova. The most famous of the professors were Averroes, Albucasis and Avenzoar. Albucasis was "the Arabian restorer of surgery. " Averroes, called in the Middle Ages "the Soul of Aristotle" or "the Commentator," is better known today among philosophers than physicians. On the revival of Moslem orthodoxy he fell upon evil days, was persecuted as a freethinker, and the saying is attributed to him—"Sit anima mea cum philosophic."

Arabian medicine had certain very definite characteristics: the basis was Greek, derived from translations of the works of Hippocrates and Galen. No contributions were made to anatomy, as dissections were prohibited, nor to physiology, and the pathology was practically that of Galen. Certain new and important diseases were described; a number of new and active remedies were introduced, chiefly from the vegetable kingdom. The Arabian hospitals were well organized and were deservedly famous. No such hospital exists today in Cairo as that which was built by al-Mansur Gilafun in 1283. The description of it by Makrizi, quoted by Neuburger,(16) reads like that of a twentieth century institution with hospital units.

(15) "I have founded this institution for my equals and for those beneath me, it is intended for rulers and subjects, for soldiers and for the emir, for great and small, freemen and slaves, men and women." "He ordered medicaments, physicians and everything else that could be required by anyone in any form of sickness; placed male and female attendants at the disposal of the patients, determined their pay, provided beds for patients and supplied them with every kind of covering that could be required in any complaint. Every class of patient was accorded separate accommodation: the four halls of the hospital were set apart for those with fever and similar complaints; one part of the building was reserved for eye-patients, one for the wounded, one for those suffering from diarrhoea, one for women; a room for convalescents was divided into two parts, one for men and one for women. Water was laid on to all these departments. One room was set apart for cooking food, preparing medicine and cooking syrups, another for the compounding of confections, balsams, eye-salves, etc. The head-physician had an apartment to himself wherein he delivered medical lectures. The number of patients was unlimited, every sick or poor person who came found admittance, nor was the duration of his stay restricted, and even those who were sick at home were supplied with every necessity."—Makrizi.

"In later times this hospital was much extended and improved. The nursing was admirable and no stint was made of drugs and appliances; each patient was provided with means upon leaving so that he should not require immediately to undertake heavy work." Neuburger: History of Medicine, Vol. 1, p. 378.

It was in the domain of chemistry that the Arabs made the greatest advances. You may remember that, in Egypt, chemistry had already made considerable strides, and I alluded to Prof. Elliot Smith's view that one of the great leaps in civilization was the discovery in the Nile Valley of the metallurgy of copper. In the brilliant period of the Ptolemies, both chemistry and pharmacology were studied, and it seems not improbable that, when the Arabs took Alexandria in the year 640, there were still many workers in these subjects.

The most famous of those early Arabic writers is the somewhat mythical Geber, who lived in the first half of the eighth century, and whose writings had an extraordinary influence throughout the Middle Ages. The whole story of Geber is discussed by Berthelot in his "La chimie au moyen age" (Paris, 1896). The transmission of Arabian science to the Occident began with the Crusades, though earlier a filtering of important knowledge in mathematics and astronomy had reached Southern and Middle Europe through Spain. Among the translators several names stand out prominently. Gerbert, who became later Pope Sylvester II, is said to have given us our present Arabic figures. You may read the story of his remarkable life in Taylor,(17) who says he was "the first mind of his time, its greatest teacher, its most eager learner, and most universal scholar." But he does not seem to have done much directly for medicine.

(17) The Mediaeval Mind, Vol. I, p. 280.

The Graeco-Arabic learning passed into Europe through two sources. As I have already mentioned, Constantinus Africanus, a North African Christian monk, widely travelled and learned in languages, came to Salernum and translated many works from Arabic into Latin, particularly those of Hippocrates and Galen. The "Pantegni" of the latter became one of the most popular textbooks of the Middle Ages. A long list of other works which he translated is given by Steinschneider.(17a) It is not unlikely that Arabic medicine had already found its way to Salernum before the time of Constantine, but the influence of his translations upon the later Middle Ages was very great.

(17a) Steinschneider: Virchow's Arch., Berl., 1867, xxxvii, 351.

The second was a more important source through the Latin translators in Spain, particularly in Toledo, where, from the middle of the twelfth till the middle of the thirteenth century, an extraordinary number of Arabic works in philosophy, mathematics and astronomy were translated. Among the translators, Gerard of Cremona is prominent, and has been called the "Father of Translators." He was one of the brightest intelligences of the Middle Ages, and did a work of the first importance to science, through the extraordinary variety of material he put in circulation. Translations, not only of the medical writers, but of an indiscriminate crowd of authors in philosophy and general literature, came from his pen. He furnished one of the first translations of the famous "Almagest" of Ptolemy, which opened the eyes of his contemporaries to the value of the Alexandrian astronomy.(18) Leclerc gives a list of seventy-one works from his hand.

(18) For an account of that remarkable work see German
    translation by Manitius, Leipzig, 1912.

Many of the translators of the period were Jews, and many of the works were translated from Hebrew into Latin. For years Arabic had been the learned language of the Jews, and in a large measure it was through them that the Arabic knowledge and the translations passed into South and Central Europe.

The Arab writer whose influence on mediaeval thought was the most profound was Averroes, the great commentator on Aristotle.

THE RISE OF THE UNIVERSITIES

THE most striking intellectual phenomenon of the thirteenth century is the rise of the universities. The story of their foundation is fully stated in Rashdall's great work (Universities of Europe in the Middle Ages, Oxford, 1895). Monastic and collegiate schools, seats of learning like Salernum, student guilds as at Bologna, had tried to meet the educational needs of the age. The word "university" literally means an association, and was not at first restricted to learned bodies. The origin appears to have been in certain guilds of students formed for mutual protection associated at some place specially favorable for study—the attraction generally being a famous teacher. The University of Bologna grew up about guilds formed by students of law, and at Paris, early in the twelfth century, there were communities of teachers, chiefly in philosophy and theology. In this way arose two different types of mediaeval university. The universities of Northern Italy were largely controlled by students, who were grouped in different "nations." They arranged the lectures and had control of the appointment of teachers. On the other hand, in the universities founded on the Paris model the masters had control of the studies, though the students, also in nations, managed their own affairs.

Two universities have a special interest at this period in connection with the development of medical studies, Bologna and Montpellier. At the former the study of anatomy was revived. In the knowledge of the structure of the human body no advance had been made for more than a thousand years—since Galen's day. In the process of translation from Greek to Syriac, from Syriac to Arabic, from Arabic to Hebrew, and from Hebrew or Arabic to Latin, both the form and thought of the old Greek writers were not infrequently confused and often even perverted, and Galen's anatomy had suffered severely in the transmission. Our earliest knowledge of the teaching of medicine at Bologna is connected with a contemporary of Dante, Taddeo Alderotti, who combined Arabian erudition with the Greek spirit. He occupied a position of extraordinary prominence, was regarded as the first citizen of Bologna and a public benefactor exempt from the payment of taxes. That he should have acquired wealth is not surprising if his usual fees were at the rate at which he charged Pope Honorius IV, i.e., two hundred florins a day, besides a "gratification" of six thousand florins.

The man who most powerfully influenced the study of medicine in Bologna was Mundinus, the first modern student of anatomy. We have seen that at the school of Salernum it was decreed that the human body should be dissected at least once every five years, but it was with the greatest difficulty that permission was obtained for this purpose. It seems probable that under the strong influence of Taddeo there was an occasional dissection at Bologna, but it was not until Mundinus (professor from 1306 to 1326) took the chair that the study of anatomy became popular. The bodies were usually those of condemned criminals, but in the year 1319 there is a record of a legal procedure against four medical students for body-snatching—the first record, as far as I know, of this gruesome practice. In 1316, Mundinus issued his work on anatomy, which served as a text-book for more than two hundred years. He quotes from Galen the amusing reasons why a man should write a book: "Firstly, to satisfy his own friends; secondly, to exercise his best mental powers; and thirdly, to be saved from the oblivion incident to old age." Scores of manuscripts of his work must have existed, but they are now excessively rare in Italy. The book was first printed at Pavia in 1478, in a small folio without figures. It was very often reprinted in the fifteenth and sixteenth centuries. The quaint illustration shows us the mediaeval method of teaching anatomy: the lecturer sitting on a chair reading from Galen, while a barber surgeon, or an "Ostensor," opens the cavities of the body.

I have already referred to the study of medicine by women at Salernum. Their names are also early met with in the school of Bologna. Mundinus is said to have had a valuable assistant, a young girl, Alessandra Giliani, an enthusiastic dissector, who was the first to practice the injection of the blood vessels with colored liquids. She died, consumed by her labors, at the early age of nineteen, and her monument is still to be seen.

Bologna honored its distinguished professors with magnificent tombs, sixteen or seventeen of which, in a wonderful state of preservation, may still be seen in the Civic Museum. That of Mundinus also exists—a sepulchral bas-relief on the wall of the Church of San Vitale at Bologna.(19)

(19) For these figures and for points relating to the old school
   at Bologna see F. G. Cavezza: Le Scuole dell' antico Studio
   Bolognese, Milano, 1896.

The other early mediaeval university of special interest in medicine is that of Montpellier. With it are connected three teachers who have left great names in our story—Arnold of Villanova, Henri de Mondeville and Guy de Chauliac. The city was very favorably situated not far from the Spanish border, and the receding tide of the Arab invasion in the eighth century had left a strong Arabic influence in that province. The date of the origin of the university is uncertain, but there were teachers of medicine there in the twelfth century, though it was not until 1289 that it was formally founded by a papal bull.

Arnold of Villanova was one of the most prolific writers of the Middle Ages. He had travelled much, was deeply read in Arabic medicine and was also a student of law and of philosophy. He was an early editor of the Regimen Sanitatis, and a strong advocate of diet and hygiene. His views on disease were largely those of the Arabian physicians, and we cannot see that he himself made any very important contribution to our knowledge; but he was a man of strong individuality and left an enduring mark on mediaeval medicine, as one may judge from the fact that among the first hundred medical books printed there were many associated with his name. He was constantly in trouble with the Church, though befriended by the Popes on account of his medical knowledge. There is a Bull of Clement V asking the bishops to search for a medical book by Arnold dedicated to himself, but not many years later his writings were condemned as heretical.

In Henri de Mondeville we have the typical mediaeval surgeon, and we know his work now very thoroughly from the editions of his "Anatomy" and "Surgery" edited by Pagel (Berlin, 1889-1892), and the fine French edition by Nicaise (Paris, 1893). The dominant Arabic influence is seen in that he quotes so large a proportion of these authors, but he was an independent observer and a practical surgeon of the first rank. He had a sharp wit and employed a bitter tongue against the medical abuses of his day. How the Hippocratic humors dominated practice at this time you may see at a glance from the table prepared by Nicaise from the works of de Mondeville. We have here the whole pathology of the period.

===
========

TABLEAU DES HUMEURS D'APRES H. DE MONDEVILLE
Flegme naturel.
F. aqueux.
Flegme   F. mucilagineux.
F. vitreux.
Flegme non naturel   F sale.
F. doux.
F. pontique, 2 especes.
F. acide, 2 especes.
Bile naturelle.
Bile   B. citrine.
B. vitelline
Bile non naturelle   B. praline.
B. aerigineuse.
B. brulee, 3 especes.
Sang   naturel.
non naturel, 5 especes.
Melancolie   naturelle.
non naturelle, 5 especes.
===
========

A still greater name in the history of this school is Guy de Chauliac, whose works have also been edited by Nicaise (Paris, 1890). His "Surgery" was one of the most important text-books of the late Middle Ages. There are many manuscripts of it, some fourteen editions in the fifteenth century and thirty-eight in the sixteenth, and it continued to be reprinted far into the seventeenth century. He too was dominated by the surgery of the Arabs, and on nearly every page one reads of the sages Avicenna, Albucasis or Rhazes. He lays down four conditions necessary for the making of a surgeon—the first is that he must be learned, the second, expert, the third that he should be clever, and the fourth that he should be well disciplined.

You will find a very discerning sketch of the relation of these two men to the history of surgery in the address given at the St. Louis Congress in 1904 by Sir Clifford Allbutt.(20) They were strong men with practical minds and good hands, whose experience taught them wisdom. In both there was the blunt honesty that so often characterizes a good surgeon, and I commend to modern surgeons de Mondeville's saying: "If you have operated conscientiously on the rich for a proper fee, and on the poor for charity, you need not play the monk, nor make pilgrimages for your soul."

(20) Allbutt: Historical Relations of Medicine and Surgery,
   London, Macmillan Co., 1905.

One other great mediaeval physician may be mentioned, Peter of Abano (a small town near Padua, famous for its baths). He is the first in a long line of distinguished physicians connected with the great school of Padua. Known as 'the Conciliator," from his attempt to reconcile the diverse views on philosophy and medicine, he had an extraordinary reputation as a practitioner and author, the persistence of which is well illustrated by the fact that eight of the one hundred and eighty-two medical books printed before 1481 were from his pen. He seems to have taught medicine in Paris, Bologna and Padua. He was a devoted astrologer, had a reputation among the people as a magician and, like his contemporary, Arnold of Villanova, came into conflict with the Church and appears to have been several times before the Inquisition; indeed it is said that he escaped the stake only by a timely death. He was a prolific commentator on Aristotle, and his exposition of the "problems" had a great vogue. The early editions of his texts are among the most superb works ever printed. He outlived his reputation as a magician, and more than a century after his death Frederick, Duke of Urbino, caused his effigies to be set up over the gate of the palace at Padua with this inscription:

PETRUS APONUS PATAVINUS
PHILOSOPHIAE MEDICINAEQUE
SCIENTISSIMUS, OB IDQUE,
CONCILIATORIS NOMEN
ADEPTUS, ASTROLOGIAE
VERO ADEO PERITUS,
UT IN MAGIAE SUSPICIONEM
INCIDERIT,
FALSOQUE DE HAERESI
POSTULATUS,
ABSOLUTUS FUERIT.(21)

(21) Naude: History of Magick, London, 1657, p. 182, or the
original: Apologie pour les grands hommes soupconnez de magic,
e.g., ed. Amst., 1719, p. 275.

It is said that Abano caused to be painted the astronomical figures in the great hall of the palace at Padua.

One characteristic of mediaeval medicine is its union with theology, which is not remarkable, as the learning of the time was chiefly in the hands of the clergy. One of the most popular works, the "Thesaurus Pauperum," was written by Petrus Hispanus, afterwards Pope John XXI. We may judge of the pontifical practice from the page here reproduced, which probably includes, under the term "iliac passion," all varieties of appendicitis.

For our purpose two beacons illuminate the spirit of the thirteenth century in its outlook on man and nature. Better than Abelard or St. Thomas Aquinas, and much better than any physicians, Albertus Magnus and Roger Bacon represent the men who were awake to greet the rising of the sun of science. What a contrast in their lives and in their works! The great Dominican's long life was an uninterrupted triumph of fruitful accomplishment—the titanic task he set himself was not only completed but was appreciated to the full by his own generation—a life not only of study and teaching, but of practical piety. As head of the order in Germany and Bishop of Regensburg, he had wide ecclesiastical influence; and in death he left a memory equalled only by one or two of his century, and excelled only by his great pupil, Thomas Aquinas. There are many Alberts in history—the Good, the Just, the Faithful—but there is only one we call "Magnus" and he richly deserved the name. What is his record? Why do we hold his name in reverence today?

Albertus Magnus was an encyclopaedic student and author, who took all knowledge for his province. His great work and his great ambition was to interpret Aristotle to his generation. Before his day, the Stagirite was known only in part, but he put within the reach of his contemporaries the whole science of Aristotle, and imbibed no small part of his spirit. He recognized the importance of the study of nature, even of testing it by way of experiment, and in the long years that had elapsed since Theophrastus no one else, except Dioscorides, had made so thorough a study of botany. His paraphrases of the natural history books of Aristotle were immensely popular, and served as a basis for all subsequent studies. Some of his medical works had an extraordinary vogue, particularly the "De Secretis Mulierum" and the "De Virtutibus Herbarum," but there is some doubt as to the authorship of the first named, although Jammy and Borgnet include it in the collected editions of his works. So fabulous was his learning that he was suspected of magic and comes in Naude's list of the wise men who have unjustly been reputed magicians. Ferguson tells(22) that "there is in actual circulation at the present time a chapbook . . . containing charms, receipts, sympathetical and magicalcures for man and animals, . . . which passes under the name of Albertus." But perhaps the greatest claim of Albertus to immortality is that he was the teacher and inspirer of Thomas Aquinas, the man who undertook the colossal task of fusing Aristotelian philosophy with Christian theology, and with such success that the "angelic doctor" remains today the supreme human authority of the Roman Catholic Church.

(22) Bibliotheca Chemica, 1906, Vol. I, p. 15.

A man of much greater interest to us from the medical point of view is Roger Bacon and for two reasons. More than any other mediaeval mind he saw the need of the study of nature by a new method. The man who could write such a sentence as this: "Experimental science has three great prerogatives over other sciences; it verifies conclusions by direct experiment; it discovers truth which they never otherwise would reach; it investigates the course of nature and opens to us a knowledge of the past and of the future," is mentally of our day and generation. Bacon was born out of due time, and his contemporaries had little sympathy with his philosophy, and still less with his mechanical schemes and inventions. From the days of the Greeks, no one had had so keen an appreciation of what experiment meant in the development of human knowledge, and he was obsessed with the idea, so commonplace to us, that knowledge should have its utility and its practical bearing. "His chief merit is that he was one of the first to point the way to original research—as opposed to the acceptance of an authority—though he himself still lacked the means of pursuing this path consistently. His inability to satisfy this impulse led to a sort of longing, which is expressed in the numerous passages in his works where he anticipates man's greater mastery over nature."(23)

(23) Dannemann: Die Naturwissenschaften in ihrer Entwicklung und
in ibrem Zusammenhange, Leipzig, 1910, Vol. I, pp. 278-279.

Bacon wrote a number of medical treatises, most of which remain in manuscript. His treatise on the "Cure of Old Age and the Preservation of Youth" was printed in English in 1683.(24) His authorities were largely Arabian. One of his manuscripts is "On the Bad Practices of Physicians." On June 10, 1914, the eve of his birth, the septencentenary of Roger Bacon will be celebrated by Oxford, the university of which he is the most distinguished ornament. His unpublished MSS. in the Bodleian will be issued by the Clarendon Press (1915-1920), and it is hoped that his unpublished medical writings will be included.

(24) It may be interesting to note the three causes to which he
    attributes old age: "As the World waxeth old, Men grow old with
    it: not by reason of the Age of the World, but because of the
    great Increase of living Creatures, which infect the very Air,
    that every way encompasseth us, and Through our Negligence in
    ordering our Lives, and That great Ignorance of the Properties
    which are in things conducing to Health, which might help a
    disordered way of Living, and might supply the defect of due
    Government."

What would have been its fate if the mind of Europe had been ready for Roger Bacon's ferment, and if men had turned to the profitable studies of physics, astronomy and chemistry instead of wasting centuries over the scholastic philosophy and the subtleties of Duns Scotus, Abelard and Thomas Aquinas? Who can say? Make no mistake about the quality of these men—giants in intellect, who have had their place in the evolution of the race; but from the standpoint of man struggling for the mastery of this world they are like the members of Swift's famous college "busy distilling sunshine from cucumbers." I speak, of course, from the position of the natural man, who sees for his fellows more hope from the experiments of Roger Bacon than from the disputations of philosophy on the "Instants, Familiarities, Quiddities and Relations," which so roused the scorn of Erasmus.

MEDIAEVAL MEDICAL STUDIES

IT will be of interest to know what studies were followed at a mediaeval university. At Oxford, as at most of the continental universities, there were three degrees, those of Bachelor, Licentiate and Doctor. The books read were the "Tegni" of Galen, the "Aphorisms" of Hippocrates, the "De Febribus" of Isaac and the "Antidotarium" of Nicolaus Salernitanus: if a graduate in arts, six years' study in all was required, in other faculties, eight. One gets very full information on such matters from a most interesting book, "Une Chaire de Medecine au XVe Siecle," by Dr. Ferrari (Paris, 1899). The University of Pavia was founded in 1361, and like most of those in Italy was largely frequented by foreigners, who were arranged, as usual, according to their nationalities; but the students do not appear to have controlled the university quite so much as at Bologna. The documents of the Ferrari family, on which the work is based, tell the story of one of its members, who was professor at Pavia from 1432 to 1472. One is surprised at the range of studies in certain directions, and still more at the absence of other subjects. A list is given of the teachers in medicine for the year 1433, twenty in all, and there were special lectures for the morning, afternoon and evening. The subjects are medicine, practical medicine, physics, metaphysics, logic, astrology, surgery and rhetoric: very striking is the omission of anatomy, which does not appear in the list even in 1467. The salaries paid were not large, so that most of the teachers must have been in practice: four hundred and five hundred florins was the maximum.

The dominance of the Arabians is striking. In 1467, special lectures were given on the "Almansor" of Rhazes, and in the catalogue of the Ferrari's library more than one half of the books are Arabian commentaries on Greek medicine. Still more striking evidence of their influence is found in the text-book of Ferrari, which was printed in 1471 and had been circulated earlier in MS. In it Avicenna is quoted more than 3000 times, Rhazes and Galen 1000, Hippocrates only 140 times. Professor Ferrari was a man who played an important role in the university, and had a large consultation practice. You will be interested to know what sort of advice he gave in special cases. I have the record of an elaborate consultation written in his own hand, from which one may gather what a formidable thing it was to fall into the hands of a mediaeval physician. Signor John de Calabria had a digestive weakness of the stomach, and rheumatic cerebral disease, combined with superfluous heat and dryness of the liver and multiplication of choler. There is first an elaborate discussion on diet and general mode of life; then he proceeds to draw up certain light medicines as a supplement, but it must have taken an extensive apothecary's shop to turn out the twenty-two prescriptions designed to meet every possible contingency.

One of the difficulties in the early days of the universities was to procure good MSS. In the Paris Faculty, the records of which are the most complete in Europe, there is an inventory for the year 1395 which gives a list of twelve volumes, nearly all by Arabian authors (25) Franklin gives an interesting incident illustrating the rarity of medical MSS. at this period. Louis XI, always worried about his health, was anxious to have in his library the works of Rhazes. The only copy available was in the library of the medical school. The manuscript was lent, but on excellent security, and it is nice to know that it was returned.

(25) Franklin: Recherches sur la Bibliotheque de la Faculte de
    Medecine de Paris, 1864.

It is said that one of the special advantages that Montpellier had over Paris was its possession of so many important MSS., particularly those of the Arabian writers. Many "Compendia" were written containing extracts from various writers, and no doubt these were extensively copied and lent or sold to students. At Bologna and Padua, there were regulations as to the price of these MSS. The university controlled the production of them, and stationers were liable to fines for inaccurate copies. The trade must have been extensive in those early days, as Rashdall mentions that in 1323 there were twenty-eight sworn booksellers in Paris, besides keepers of bookstalls in the open air.

MEDIAEVAL PRACTICE

THE Greek doctrine of the four humors colored all the conceptions of disease; upon their harmony alone it was thought that health depended. The four temperaments, sanguine, phlegmatic, bilious and melancholic, corresponded with the prevalence of these humors. The body was composed of certain so-called "naturals," seven in number—the elements, the temperaments, the humors, the members or parts, the virtues or faculties, the operations or functions and the spirits. Certain "non-naturals," nine in number, preserved the health of the body, viz. air, food and drink, movement and repose, sleeping and waking, excretion and retention, and the passions. Disease was due usually to alterations in the composition of the humors, and the indications for treatment were in accordance with these doctrines. They were to be evacuated, tenuated, cooled, heated, purged or strengthened. This humoral doctrine prevailed throughout the Middle Ages, and reached far into modern times—indeed, echoes of it are still to be heard in popular conversations on the nature of disease.

The Arabians were famous for their vigor and resource in matters of treatment. Bleeding was the first resort in a large majority of all diseases. In the "Practice" of Ferrari there is scarcely a malady for which it is not recommended. All remedies were directed to the regulation of the six non-naturals, and they either preserved health, cured the disease or did the opposite. The most popular medicines were derived from the vegetable kingdom, and as they were chiefly those recommended by Galen, they were, and still are, called by his name. Many important mineral medicines were introduced by the Arabians, particularly mercury, antimony, iron, etc. There were in addition scores of substances, the parts or products of animals, some harmless, others salutary, others again useless and disgusting. Minor surgery was in the hands of the barbers, who performed all the minor operations, such as bleeding; the more important operations, few in number, were performed by surgeons.

ASTROLOGY AND DIVINATION

AT this period astrology, which included astronomy, was everywhere taught. In the "Gouernaunce of Prynces, or Pryvete of Pryveties," translated by James Yonge, 1422,(26) there occurs the statement: "As Galian the lull wies leche Saith and Isoder the Gode clerk, hit witnessith that a man may not perfitely can the sciens and craft of Medissin but yef he be an astronomoure."

(26) Early English Text Society, Extra Series, No. LXXIV, p. 195, 1898; Secreta Secretorum, Rawl. MS. B., 490.

We have seen how the practice of astrology spread from Babylonia and Greece throughout the Roman Empire. It was carried on into the Middle Ages as an active and aggressive cult, looked upon askance at times by the Church, but countenanced by the courts, encouraged at the universities, and always by the public. In the curriculum of the mediaeval university, astronomy made up with music, arithmetic and geometry the Quadrivium. In the early faculties, astronomy and astrology were not separate, and at Bologna, in the early fourteenth century, we meet with a professorship of astrology.(27) One of the duties of this salaried professor, was to supply "judgements" gratis for the benefit of enquiring students, a treacherous and delicate assignment, as that most distinguished occupant of the chair at Bologna, Cecco d'Ascoli, found when he was burned at the stake in 1357, a victim of the Florentine Inquisition.(28)

(27) Rashdall: Universities of Europe in the Middle Ages, Vol. I, p. 240.

(28) Rashdall, l.c., Vol. I, p. 244.—Rashdall also mentions that
in the sixteenth century at Oxford there is an instance of a
scholar admitted to practice astrology. l.c., Vol. II, p. 458.

Roger Bacon himself was a warm believer in judicial astrology and in the influence of the planets, stars and comets on generation, disease and death.

Many of the stronger minds of the Renaissance broke away from the follies of the subject. Thus Cornelius Agrippa in reply to the request of a friar to consult the stars on his behalf says:(29) "Judicial astrology is nothing more than the fallacious guess of superstitious men, who have founded a science on uncertain things and are deceived by it: so think nearly all the wise; as such it is ridiculed by some most noble philosophers; Christian theologians reject it, and it is condemned by sacred councils of the Church. Yet you, whose office it is to dissuade others from these vanities, oppressed, or rather blinded by I know not what distress of mind, flee to this as to a sacred augur, and as if there were no God in Israel, that you send to inquire of the god of Ekron."

(29) H. Morley: The Life of Henry Cornelius Agrippa, London, 1856, Vol. II, p. 138.

In spite of the opposition of the Church astrology held its own; many of the universities at the end of the fifteenth century published almanacs, usually known as "Prognosticons," and the practice was continued far into the sixteenth century. I show you here an illustration. Rabelais, you may remember, when physician to the Hotel Dieu in Lyons, published almanacs for the years 1533, 1535, 1541, 1546. In the title-page he called himself "Doctor of Medicine and Professor of Astrology," and they continued to be printed under his name until 1556. In the preparation of these he must have had his tongue in his cheek, as in his famous "Pantagrueline Prognostication," in which, to satisfy the curiosity of all good companions, he had turned over all the archives of the heavens, calculated the quadratures of the moon, hooked out all that has ever been thought by all the Astrophils, Hypernephilists, Anemophylakes, Uranopets and Ombrophori, and felt on every point with Empedocles.(30)

(30) Pantagrueline Prognostication, Rabelais, W. F. Smith's
 translation, 1893, Vol. II, p. 460.

Even physicians of the most distinguished reputation practised judicial astrology. Jerome Cardan was not above earning money by casting horoscopes, and on this subject he wrote one of his most popular books (De Supplemento Almanach, etc., 1543), in which astronomy and astrology are mixed in the truly mediaeval fashion. He gives in it some sixty-seven nativities, remarkable for the events they foretell, with an exposition. One of the accusations brought against him was that he had "attempted to subject to the stars the Lord of the stars and cast our Saviour's horoscope."(31) Cardan professed to have abandoned a practice looked upon with disfavor both by the Church and by the universities, but he returned to it again and again. I show here his own horoscope. That remarkable character, Michael Servetus, the discoverer of the lesser circulation, when a fellow student with Vesalius at Paris, gave lectures upon judicial astrology, which brought him into conflict with the faculty; and the rarest of the Servetus works, rarer even than the "Christianismi Restitutio," is the "Apologetica disceptatio pro astrologia," one copy of which is in the Bibliotheque Nationale. Nor could the new astronomy and the acceptance of the heliocentric views dislocate the popular belief. The literature of the seventeenth century is rich in astrological treatises dealing with medicine.

(31) De Thou, Lib. LXII, quoted by Morley in Life of Jerome
 Cardan, Vol. II, p. 294.

No one has ever poured such satire upon the mantic arts as did Rabelais in chapter twenty-five of the third book of "Pantagruel." Panurge goes to consult Her Trippa—the famous Cornelius Agrippa, whose opinion of astrology has already been quoted, but who nevertheless, as court astrologer to Louise of Savoy, had a great contemporary reputation. After looking Panurge in the face and making conclusions by metoposcopy and physiognomy, he casts his horoscope secundum artem, then, taking a branch of tamarisk, a favorite tree from which to get the divining rod, he names some twenty-nine or thirty mantic arts, from pyromancy to necromancy, by which he offers to predict his future. While full of rare humor, this chapter throws an interesting light on the extraordinary number of modes of divination that have been employed. Small wonder that Panurge repented of his visit! I show here the title-page of a popular book by one of the most famous of the English astrological physicians, Nicholas Culpeper.

Never was the opinion of sensible men on this subject better expressed than by Sir Thomas Browne:(32) "Nor do we hereby reject or condemn a sober and regulated Astrology; we hold there is more truth therein than in ASTROLOGERS; in some more than many allow, yet in none so much as some pretend. We deny not the influence of the Starres, but often suspect the due application thereof; for though we should affirm that all things were in all things; that Heaven were but Earth Celestified, and earth but Heaven terrestrified, or that each part above had an influence upon its divided affinity below; yet how to single out these relations, and duly to apply their actions, is a work ofttimes to be effected by some revelation, and Cabala from above, rather than any Philosophy, or speculation here below."

(32) Sir Thomas Browne:
Pseudodoxia Epidemica, Bk. IV, Chap.
 XIII. (Wilkin's ed., Vol. III, p. 84.)

As late as 1699, a thesis was discussed at the Paris Faculty, "Whether comets were harbingers of disease," and in 1707 the Faculty negatived the question propounded in a thesis, "Whether the moon had any sway on the human body."

The eighteenth and nineteenth centuries saw, among intelligent men, a progressive weakening of the belief in the subject; but not even the satire of Swift, with his practical joke in predicting and announcing the death of the famous almanac maker, nor contemptuous neglect of the subject of late years sufficed to dispel the belief from the minds of the public. Garth in the Dispensary (1699) satirizes the astrological practitioners of his day:

The Sage in Velvet Chair, here lolls at Ease
To promise future Health for present Fees
Then as from Tripod solemn Sham reveals
And what the Stars know nothing of foretell. (Canto ii.)

The almanacs of Moore and Zadkiel continue to be published, and remain popular. In London, sandwich men are to be met with carrying advertisements of Chaldeans and Egyptians who offer to tell your fortune by the stars. Even in this country, astrology is still practiced to a surprising extent if one may judge from advertisements in certain papers, and from publications which must have a considerable sale. Many years ago, I had as a patient an estimable astrologer, whose lucrative income was derived from giving people astral information as to the rise and fall of stocks. It is a chapter in the vagaries of the human mind that is worth careful study.(33) Let me commend to your reading the sympathetic story called "A Doctor of Medicine" in the "Rewards and Fairies" of Kipling. The hero is Nicholas Culpeper, Gent., whose picture is here given. One stanza of the poem at the end of the story, "Our Fathers of Old," may be quoted:

> Wonderful tales had our fathers of old—
> Wonderful tales of the herbs and the stars—
> The Sun was Lord of the Marigold,
> Basil and Rocket belonged to Mars.
> Pat as a sum in division it goes—
> (Every plant had a star bespoke)—
> Who but Venus should govern the Rose?
> Who but Jupiter own the Oak?
> Simply and gravely the facts are told
> In the wonderful books of our fathers of old.

(33) It is not generally known that Stonewall Jackson practiced astrology. Col. J. W. Revere in "Keel and Saddle" (Boston, 1872) tells of meeting Jackson in 1852 on a Mississippi steamer and talking with him on the subject. Some months later, Revere received a letter from Jackson enclosing his (Revere's) horoscope. There was a "culmination of the malign aspect during the first days of May, 1863—both will be exposed to a common danger at the time indicated." At the battle of Chancellorsville, May 9, 1863, Revere saw Jackson mortally wounded!

James J. Walsh of New York has written a book of extraordinary interest called "The Thirteenth, Greatest of Centuries." I have not the necessary knowledge to say whether he has made out his case or not for art and for literature. There was certainly a great awakening and, inspired by high ideals, men turned with a true instinct to the belief that there was more in life than could be got out of barren scholastic studies. With many of the strong men of the period one feels the keenest mental sympathy. Grosseteste, the great Clerk of Lincoln, as a scholar, a teacher and a reformer, represents a type of mind that could grow only in fruitful soil. Roger Bacon may be called the first of the moderns—certainly the first to appreciate the extraordinary possibilities which lay in a free and untrammelled study of nature. A century which could produce men capable of building the Gothic cathedrals may well be called one of the great epochs in history, and the age that produced Dante is a golden one in literature. Humanity has been the richer for St. Francis; and Abelard, Albertus and Aquinas form a trio not easy to match, in their special departments, either before or after. But in science, and particularly in medicine, and in the advance of an outlook upon nature, the thirteenth century did not help man very much. Roger Bacon was "a voice crying in the wilderness," and not one of the men I have picked out as specially typical of the period instituted any new departure either in practice or in science. They were servile followers, when not of the Greeks, of the Arabians. This is attested by the barrenness of the century and a half that followed. One would have thought that the stimulus given by Mundinus to the study of anatomy would have borne fruit, but little was done in science during the two and a half centuries that followed the delivery of his lectures and still less in the art. While William of Wykeham was building Winchester Cathedral and Chaucer was writing the Canterbury Tales, John of Gaddesden in practice was blindly following blind leaders whose authority no one dared question.

The truth is, from the modern standpoint the thirteenth was not the true dawn brightening more and more unto the perfect day, but a glorious aurora which flickered down again into the arctic night of mediaevalism.

To sum up—in medicine the Middle Ages represent a restatement from century to century of the facts and theories of the Greeks modified here and there by Arabian practice. There was, in Francis Bacon's phrase, much iteration, small addition. The schools bowed in humble, slavish submission to Galen and Hippocrates, taking everything from them but their spirit and there was no advance in our knowledge of the structure or function of the body. The Arabians lit a brilliant torch from Grecian lamps and from the eighth to the eleventh centuries the profession reached among them a position of dignity and importance to which it is hard to find a parallel in history.

CHAPTER IV — THE RENAISSANCE AND THE RISE OF ANATOMY AND PHYSIOLOGY

THE "reconquest of the classic world of thought was by far the most important achievement of the fifteenth and sixteenth centuries. It absorbed nearly the whole mental energy of the Italians. The revelation of what men were and what they wrought under the influence of other faiths and other impulses, in distant ages with a different ideal for their aim, not only widened the narrow horizon of the Middle Ages, but it also restored self-confidence to the reason of humanity."(1)

(1) J. A. Symonds: The Renaissance in Italy; the Revival of Learning, 1877, p. 52.

Everywhere throughout the Middle Ages learning was the handmaid of theology. Even Roger Bacon with his strong appeal for a new method accepted the dominant mediaeval conviction—that all the sciences did but minister to their queen, Theology. A new spirit entered man's heart as he came to look upon learning as a guide to the conduct of life. A revolution was slowly effected in the intellectual world. It is a mistake to think of the Renaissance as a brief period of sudden fruitfulness in the North Italian cities. So far as science is concerned, the thirteenth century was an aurora followed by a long period of darkness, but the fifteenth was a true dawn that brightened more and more unto the perfect day. Always a reflex of its period, medicine joined heartily though slowly in the revolt against mediaevalism. How slowly I did not appreciate until recently. Studying the earliest printed medical works to catch the point of view of the men who were in the thick of the movement up to 1480—which may be taken to include the first quarter of a century of printing—one gets a startling record. The mediaeval mind still dominates: of the sixty-seven authors of one hundred and eighty-two editions of early medical books, twenty-three were men of the thirteenth and fourteenth centuries, thirty men of the fifteenth century, eight wrote in Arabic, several were of the School of Salernum, and only six were of classical antiquity, viz., Pliny (first 1469), Hippocrates (1473) (Hain (*)7247), Galen (1475) (Hain 7237), Aristotle (1476), Celsus (1478), and Dioscorides (1478).(**)

(*) This asterisk is used by Hain to indicate that he had seen a
   copy.—Ed.

(**) Data added to a manuscript taken from the author's summary
   on "Printed Medical Books to 1480" in Transactions of the
   Bibliographical Society, London, 1916, XIII, 5-8, revised from
   its "News-Sheet" (February, 1914). "Of neither Hippocrates nor
   Galen is there an early edition; but in 1473 at Pavia appeared an
   exposition of the Aphorisms of Hippocrates, and in 1475 at Padua
   an edition of the Tegni or Notes of Galen." Ibid., p. 6.
   Osler's unfinished Illustrated Monograph on this subject is now
   being printed for the Society of which he was President.—Ed.

The medical profession gradually caught the new spirit. It has been well said that Greece arose from the dead with the New Testament in the one hand and Aristotle in the other. There was awakened a perfect passion for the old Greek writers, and with it a study of the original sources, which had now become available in many manuscripts. Gradually Hippocrates and Galen came to their own again. Almost every professor of medicine became a student of the MSS. of Aristotle and of the Greek physicians, and before 1530 the presses had poured out a stream of editions. A wave of enthusiasm swept over the profession, and the best energies of its best minds were devoted to a study of the Fathers. Galen became the idol of the schools. A strong revulsion of feeling arose against the Arabians, and Avicenna, the Prince, who had been clothed with an authority only a little less than divine, became anathema. Under the leadership of the Montpellier School, the Arabians made a strong fight, but it was a losing battle all along the line. This group of medical humanists—men who were devoted to the study of the old humanities, as Latin and Greek were called—has had a great and beneficial influence upon the profession. They were for the most part cultivated gentlemen with a triple interest—literature, medicine and natural history. How important is the part they played may be gathered from a glance at the "Lives" given by Bayle in his "Biographic Medicale" (Paris, 1855) between the years 1500 and 1575. More than one half of them had translated or edited works of Hippocrates or Galen; many of them had made important contributions to general literature, and a large proportion of them were naturalists: Leonicenus, Linacre, Champier, Fernel, Fracastorius, Gonthier, Caius, J. Sylvius, Brasavola, Fuchsius, Matthiolus, Conrad Gesner, to mention only those I know best, form a great group. Linacre edited Greek works for Aldus, translated works of Galen, taught Greek at Oxford, wrote Latin grammars and founded the Royal College of Physicians.(*) Caius was a keen Greek scholar, an ardent student of natural history, and his name is enshrined as co-founder of one of the most important of the Cambridge colleges. Gonthier, Fernel, Fuchs and Mattioli were great scholars and greater physicians. Champier, one of the most remarkable of the group, was the founder of the Hotel Dieu at Lyons, and author of books of a characteristic Renaissance type and of singular bibliographical interest. In many ways greatest of all was Conrad Gesner, whose mors inopinata at forty-nine, bravely fighting the plague, is so touchingly and tenderly mourned by his friend Caius. (2) Physician, botanist, mineralogist, geologist, chemist, the first great modern bibliographer, he is the very embodiment of the spirit of the age.(2a) On the flyleaf of my copy of the "Bibliotheca Universalis" (1545), is written a fine tribute to his memory. I do not know by whom it is, but I do know from my reading that it is true:

(*) Cf. Osler: Thomas Linacre, Cambridge University Press,
   1908.—Ed.

(2) Joannis Caii Britanni de libris suis, etc., 1570.

(2a) See J. C. Bay: Papers Bibliog. Soc. of America, 1916, X,
   No. 2, 53-86.

"Conrad Gesner, who kept open house there for all learned men who came into his neighborhood. Gesner was not only the best naturalist among the scholars of his day, but of all men of that century he was the pattern man of letters. He was faultless in private life, assiduous in study, diligent in maintaining correspondence and good-will with learned men in all countries, hospitable—though his means were small—to every scholar that came into Zurich. Prompt to serve all, he was an editor of other men's volumes, a writer of prefaces for friends, a suggestor to young writers of books on which they might engage themselves, and a great helper to them in the progress of their work. But still, while finding time for services to other men, he could produce as much out of his own study as though he had no part in the life beyond its walls."

A large majority of these early naturalists and botanists were physicians. (3) The Greek art of observation was revived in a study of the scientific writings of Aristotle, Theophrastus and Dioscorides and in medicine, of Hippocrates and of Galen, all in the Greek originals. That progress was at first slow was due in part to the fact that the leaders were too busy scraping the Arabian tarnish from the pure gold of Greek medicine and correcting the anatomical mistakes of Galen to bother much about his physiology or pathology. Here and there among the great anatomists of the period we read of an experiment, but it was the art of observation, the art of Hippocrates, not the science of Galen, not the carefully devised experiment to determine function, that characterized their work. There was indeed every reason why men should have been content with the physiology and pathology of that day, as, from a theoretical standpoint, it was excellent. The doctrine of the four humors and of the natural, animal and vital spirits afforded a ready explanation for the symptoms of all diseases, and the practice of the day was admirably adapted to the theories. There was no thought of, no desire for, change. But the revival of learning awakened in men at first a suspicion and at last a conviction that the ancients had left something which could be reached by independent research, and gradually the paralytic-like torpor passed away.

(3) Miall: The Early Naturalists, London, 1912.

The sixteenth and seventeenth centuries did three things in medicine—shattered authority, laid the foundation of an accurate knowledge of the structure of the human body and demonstrated how its functions should be studied intelligently—with which advances, as illustrating this period, may be associated the names of Paracelsus, Vesalius and Harvey.

PARACELSUS

PARACELSUS is "der Geist der stets verneint." He roused men against the dogmatism of the schools, and he stimulated enormously the practical study of chemistry. These are his great merits, against which must be placed a flood of hermetical and transcendental medicine, some his own, some foisted in his name, the influence of which is still with us.

"With what judgment ye judge it shall be judged to you again" is the verdict of three centuries on Paracelsus. In return for unmeasured abuse of his predecessors and contemporaries he has been held up to obloquy as the arch-charlatan of history. We have taken a cheap estimate of him from Fuller and Bacon, and from a host of scurrilous scribblers who debased or perverted his writings. Fuller(4) picked him out as exemplifying the drunken quack, whose body was a sea wherein the tide of drunkenness was ever ebbing and flowing—"He boasted that shortly he would order Luther and the Pope, as well as he had done Galen and Hippocrates. He was never seen to pray, and seldome came to Church. He was not onely skilled in naturall Magick (the utmost bounds whereof border on the suburbs of hell) but is charged to converse constantly with familiars. Guilty he was of all vices but wantonnesse: . . . "

(4) Fuller: The Holy and Profane State, Cambridge, 1642, p. 56.

Francis Bacon, too, says many hard things of him.(5)

(5) Bacon: Of the Proficience and Advancement of Learning, Bk.
II, Pickering ed., London, 1840, p. 181. Works, Spedding ed.,
III, 381.

To the mystics, on the other hand, he is Paracelsus the Great, the divine, the most supreme of the Christian magi, whose writings are too precious for science, the monarch of secrets, who has discovered the Universal Medicine. This is illustrated in Browning's well-known poem "Paracelsus," published when he was only twenty-one; than which there is no more pleasant picture in literature of the man and of his aspirations. His was a "searching and impetuous soul" that sought to win from nature some startling secret—". . . a tincture of force to flush old age with youth, or breed gold, or imprison moonbeams till they change to opal shafts!" At the same time with that capacity for self-deception which characterizes the true mystic he sought to cast

Light on a darkling race; save for that doubt,
I stood at first where all aspire at last
To stand: the secret of the world was mine.
I knew, I felt (perception unexpressed,
Uncomprehended by our narrow thought,
But somehow felt and known in every shift
And change in the spirit,—nay, in every pore
Of the body, even)—what God is, what we are,
What life is—. . .(6)

(6) Robert Browning: Paracelsus, closing speech.

Much has been done of late to clear up his story and his character. Professor Sudhoff, of Leipzig, has made an exhaustive bibliographical study of his writings,(7) there have been recent monographs by Julius Hartmann, and Professors Franz and Karl Strunz,(8) and a sympathetic summary of his life and writings has been published by the late Miss Stoddart.(9) Indeed there is at present a cult of Paracelsus. The hermetic and alchemical writings are available in English in the edition of A. E. Waite, London, 1894. The main facts of his life you can find in all the biographies. Suffice it here to say that he was born at Einsiedeln, near Zurich, in 1493, the son of a physician, from whom he appears to have had his early training both in medicine and in chemistry. Under the famous abbot and alchemist, Trithemius of Wurzburg, he studied chemistry and occultism. After working in the mines at Schwatz he began his wanderings, during which he professes to have visited nearly all the countries in Europe and to have reached India and China. Returning to Germany he began a triumphal tour of practice through the German cities, always in opposition to the medical faculty, and constantly in trouble. He undoubtedly performed many important cures, and was thought to have found the supreme secret of alchemistry. In the pommel of his sword he was believed to carry a familiar spirit. So dominant was his reputation that in 1527 he was called to the chair of physic in the University of Basel. Embroiled in quarrels after his first year he was forced to leave secretly, and again began his wanderings through German cities, working, quarrelling, curing, and dying prematurely at Saltzburg in 1541—one of the most tragic figures in the history of medicine.

(7) Professor Sudhoff:
Bibliographia Paracelsica, Berlin, 1894,
    1899.

(8) R. Julius Hartmann: Theophrast von Hohenheim, Berlin, 1904;
    ditto, Franz Strunz, Leipzig, 1903.

(9) Anna M. Stoddart: The Life of Paracelsus, London, John
    Murray, 1911.

Paracelsus is the Luther of medicine, the very incarnation of the spirit of revolt. At a period when authority was paramount, and men blindly followed old leaders, when to stray from the beaten track in any field of knowledge was a damnable heresy, he stood out boldly for independent study and the right of private judgment. After election to the chair at Basel he at once introduced a startling novelty by lecturing in German. He had caught the new spirit and was ready to burst all bonds both in medicine and in theology. He must have startled the old teachers and practitioners by his novel methods. "On June 5, 1527, he attached a programme of his lectures to the black-board of the University inviting all to come to them. It began by greeting all students of the art of healing. He proclaimed its lofty and serious nature, a gift of God to man, and the need of developing it to new importance and to new renown. This he undertook to do, not retrogressing to the teaching of the ancients, but progressing whither nature pointed, through research into nature, where he himself had discovered and had verified by prolonged experiment and experience. He was ready to oppose obedience to old lights as if they were oracles from which one did not dare to differ. Illustrious doctor might be graduated from books, but books made not a single physician.(10) Neither graduation, nor fluency, nor the knowledge of old languages, nor the reading of many books made a physician, but the knowledge of things themselves and their properties. The business of a doctor was to know the different kinds of sicknesses, their causes, their symptoms and their right remedies. This he would teach, for he had won this knowledge through experience, the greatest teacher, and with much toil. He would teach it as he had learned it, and his lectures would be founded on works which he had composed concerning inward and external treatment, physic and surgery."(11) Shortly afterwards, at the Feast of St. John, the students had a bonfire in front of the university. Paracelsus came out holding in his hands the "Bible of medicine," Avicenna's "Canon," which he flung into the flames saying: "Into St. John's fire so that all misfortune may go into the air with the smoke." It was, as he explained afterwards, a symbolic act: "What has perished must go to the fire; it is no longer fit for use: what is true and living, that the fire cannot burn." With abundant confidence in his own capacity he proclaimed himself the legitimate monarch, the very Christ of medicine. "You shall follow me," cried he, "you, Avicenna, Galen, Rhasis, Montagnana, Mesues; you, Gentlemen of Paris, Montpellier, Germany, Cologne, Vienna, and whomsoever the Rhine and Danube nourish; you who inhabit the isles of the sea; you, likewise, Dalmatians, Athenians; thou, Arab; thou, Greek; thou, Jew; all shall follow me, and the monarchy shall be mine."(12)

(10) And men have oft grown old among their books
To die case hardened in their ignorance.

—Paracelsus, Browning.

(11) Anna M. Stoddart: Life of Paracelsus, London, 1911, pp. 95-96.

(12) Browning's Paracelsus, London, 1835, p. 206 (note).

This first great revolt against the slavish authority of the schools had little immediate effect, largely on account of the personal vagaries of the reformer—but it made men think. Paracelsus stirred the pool as had not been done for fifteen centuries.

Much more important is the relation of Paracelsus to the new chemical studies, and their relation to practical medicine. Alchemy, he held, "is to make neither gold nor silver: its use is to make the supreme sciences and to direct them against disease." He recognized three basic substances, sulphur, mercury and salt, which were the necessary ingredients of all bodies organic or inorganic. They were the basis of the three principles out of which the Archaeus, the spirit of nature, formed all bodies. He made important discoveries in chemistry; zinc, the various compounds of mercury, calomel, flowers of sulphur, among others, and he was a strong advocate of the use of preparations of iron and antimony. In practical pharmacy he has perhaps had a greater reputation for the introduction of a tincture of opium—labdanum or laudanum—with which he effected miraculous cures, and the use of which he had probably learned in the East.

Through Paracelsus a great stimulus was given to the study of chemistry and pharmacy, and he is the first of the modern iatro-chemists. In contradistinction to Galenic medicines, which were largely derived from the vegetable kingdom, from this time on we find in the literature references to spagyric medicines and a "spagyrist" was a Paracelsian who regarded chemistry as the basis of all medical knowledge.

One cannot speak very warmly of the practical medical writings of Paracelsus. Gout, which may be taken as the disease upon which he had the greatest reputation, is very badly described, and yet he has one or two fruitful ideas singularly mixed with mediaeval astrology; but he has here and there very happy insights, as where he remarks "nec praeter synoviam locqum alium ullum podagra occupat."(13) In the tract on phlebotomy I see nothing modern, and here again he is everywhere dominated by astrological ideas—"Sapiens dominatur astris."

(13) Geneva ed., 1658, Vol. I, p. 613.

As a protagonist of occult philosophy, Paracelsus has had a more enduring reputation than as a physician. In estimating his position there is the great difficulty referred to by Sudhoff in determining which of the extant treatises are genuine. In the two volumes issued in English by Waite in 1894, there is much that is difficult to read and to appreciate from our modern standpoint. In the book "Concerning Long Life" he confesses that his method and practice will not be intelligible to common persons and that he writes only for those whose intelligence is above the average. To those fond of transcendental studies they appeal and are perhaps intelligible. Everywhere one comes across shrewd remarks which prove that Paracelsus had a keen belief in the all-controlling powers of nature and of man's capacity to make those powers operate for his own good: "the wise man rules Nature, not Nature the wise man." "The difference between the Saint and the Magus is that the one operates by means of God, and the other by means of Nature. " He had great faith in nature and the light of nature, holding that man obtains from nature according as he believes. His theory of the three principles appears to have controlled his conception of everything relating to man, spiritually, mentally and bodily; and his threefold genera of disease corresponded in some mysterious way with the three primary substances, salt, sulphur and mercury.

How far he was a believer in astrology, charms and divination it is not easy to say. From many of the writings in his collected works one would gather, as I have already quoted, that he was a strong believer. On the other hand, in the "Paramirum," he says: "Stars control nothing in us, suggest nothing, incline to nothing, own nothing; they are free from us and we are free from them" (Stoddart, p. 185). The Archaeus, not the stars, controls man's destiny. "Good fortune comes from ability, and ability comes from the spirit" (Archaeus).

No one has held more firmly the dualistic conception of the healing art. There are two kinds of doctors; those who heal miraculously and those who heal through medicine. Only he who believes can work miracles. The physician has to accomplish that which God would have done miraculously, had there been faith enough in the sick man (Stoddart, p. 194). He had the Hippocratic conception of the "vis medicatrix naturae"—no one keener since the days of the Greeks. Man is his own doctor and finds proper healing herbs in his own garden: the physician is in ourselves, in our own nature are all things that we need: and speaking of wounds, with singular prescience he says that the treatment should be defensive so that no contingency from without could hinder Nature in her work (Stoddart, p. 213).

Paracelsus expresses the healing powers of nature by the word "mumia," which he regarded as a sort of magnetic influence or force, and he believed that anyone possessing this could arrest or heal disease in others. As the lily breaks forth in invisible perfume, so healing influences may pass from an invisible body. Upon these views of Paracelsus was based the theory of the sympathetic cure of disease which had an extraordinary vogue in the late sixteenth and seventeenth centuries, and which is not without its modern counterpart.

In the next century, in Van Helmont we meet with the Archaeus everywhere presiding, controlling and regulating the animate and inanimate bodies, working this time through agents, local ferments. The Rosicrucians had their direct inspiration from his writings, and such mystics as the English Rosicrucian Fludd were strong Paracelsians.(14)

(14) Robert Fludd, the Mystical Physician, British Medical Journal, London, 1897, ii, 408.

The doctrine of contraries drawn from the old Greek philosophy, upon which a good deal of the treatment of Hippocrates and Galen was based—dryness expelled by moisture, cold by heat, etc. —was opposed by Paracelsus in favor of a theory of similars, upon which the practice of homeopathy is based. This really arose from the primitive beliefs, to which I have already referred as leading to the use of eyebright in diseases of the eye, and cyclamen in diseases of the ear because of its resemblance to that part; and the Egyptian organotherapy had the same basis,—spleen would cure spleen, heart, heart, etc. In the sixteenth and seventeenth centuries these doctrines of sympathies and antipathies were much in vogue. A Scotchman, Sylvester Rattray, edited in the "Theatrum Sympatheticum"(15) all the writings upon the sympathies and antipathies of man with animal, vegetable and mineral substances, and the whole art of physics was based on this principle.

(15) Rattray: Theatrum Sympatheticum, Norimberge, MDCLXII.

Upon this theory of "mumia," or magnetic force, the sympathetic cure of disease was based. The weapon salve, the sympathetic ointment, and the famous powder of sympathy were the instruments through which it acted. The magnetic cure of wounds became the vogue. Van Helmont adopted these views in his famous treatise "De Magnetica Vulnerum Curatione,"(16) in which he asserted that cures were wrought through magnetic influence. How close they came to modern views of wound infection may be judged from the following: "Upon the solution of Unity in any part the ambient air . . . repleted with various evaporations or aporrhoeas of mixt bodies, especially such as are then suffering the act of putrefaction, violently invadeth the part and thereupon impresseth an exotic miasm or noxious diathesis, which disposeth the blood successively arriving at the wound, to putrefaction, by the intervention of fermentation." With his magnetic sympathy, Van

Helmont expressed clearly the doctrine of immunity and the cure of disease by immune sera: "For he who has once recovered from that disease hath not only obtained a pure balsaamical blood, whereby for the future he is rendered free from any recidivation of the same evil, but also infallibly cures the same affection in his neighbour . . . and by the mysterious power of Magnetism transplants that balsaam and conserving quality into the blood of another." He was rash enough to go further and say that the cures effected by the relics of the saints were also due to the same cause—a statement which led to a great discussion with the theologians and to Van Helmont's arrest for heresy, and small wonder, when he makes such bold statements as "Let the Divine enquire only concerning God, the Naturalist concerning Nature," and "God in the production of miracles does for the most part walk hand in hand with Nature."

(16) An English translation by Walter Charleton appeared in 1650, entitled "A Ternary of Paradoxes."

That wandering genius, Sir Kenelm Digby, did much to popularize this method of treatment by his lecture on the "Powder of Sympathy."(17) His powder was composed of copperas alone or mixed with gum tragacanth. He regarded the cure as effected through the subtle influence of the sympathetic spirits or, as Highmore says, by "atomicall energy wrought at a distance," and the remedy could be applied to the wound itself, or to a cloth soaked in the blood or secretions, or to the weapon that caused the wound. One factor leading to success may have been that in the directions which Digby gave for treating the wound (in the celebrated case of James Howell, for instance), it was to be let alone and kept clean. The practice is alluded to very frequently by the poets. In the "Lay of the Last Minstrel" we find the following:

(17) French edition, 1668, English translation, same year. For a
   discussion on the author of the weapon salve see Van Helmont, who

gives the various formulas. Highmore (1651) says the "powder is
   a Zaphyrian salt calcined by a celestial fire operating in Leo
   and Cancer into a Lunar complexion."

But she has ta'en the broken lance,
And wash'd it from the clotted gore,
And salved the splinter o'er and o'er.
William of Deloraine, in trance,
Whene'er she turn'd it round and round,
Twisted, as if she gall'd his wound,
Then to her maidens she did say,
That he should be whole man and sound,

(Canto iii, xxiii.)

and in Dryden's "Tempest" (V, 1) Ariel says:

Anoint the Sword which pierc'd him with the Weapon-Salve,
   And wrap it close from Air till I have time
To visit him again.

From Van Helmont comes the famous story of the new nose that dropped off in sympathy with the dead arm from which it was taken, and the source of the famous lines of Hudibras. As I have not seen the original story quoted of late years it may be worth while to give it: "A certain inhabitant of Bruxels, in a combat had his nose mowed off, addressed himself to Tagliacozzus, a famous Chirurgeon, living at Bononia, that he might procure a new one; and when he feared the incision of his own arm, he hired a Porter to admit it, out of whose arm, having first given the reward agreed upon, at length he dig'd a new nose. About thirteen moneths after his return to his own Countrey, on a sudden the ingrafted nose grew cold, putrified, and within few days drops off. To those of his friends that were curious in the exploration of the cause of this unexpected misfortune, it was discovered, that the Porter expired, neer about the same punctilio of time, wherein the nose grew frigid and cadaverous. There

are at Bruxels yet surviving, some of good repute, that were eye-witnesses of these occurrences."(18)

(18) Charleton: Of the Magnetic Cure of Wounds, London, 1650, p. 13.

Equally in the history of science and of medicine, 1542 is a starred year, marked by a revolution in our knowledge alike of Macrocosm and Microcosm. In Frauenburg, the town physician and a canon, now nearing the Psalmist limit and his end, had sent to the press the studies of a lifetime—"De revolutionibus orbium coelestium." It was no new thought, no new demonstration that Copernicus thus gave to his generation. Centuries before, men of the keenest scientific minds from Pythagoras on had worked out a heliocentric theory, fully promulgated by Aristarchus, and very generally accepted by the brilliant investigators of the Alexandrian school; but in the long interval, lapped in Oriental lethargy, man had been content to acknowledge that the heavens declare the glory of God and that the firmament sheweth his handiwork. There had been great astronomers before Copernicus. In the fifteenth century Nicholas of Cusa and Regiomontanus had hinted at the heliocentric theory; but 1512 marks an epoch in the history of science, since for all time Copernicus put the problem in a way that compelled acquiescence.

Nor did Copernicus announce a truth perfect and complete, not to be modified, but there were many contradictions and lacunae which the work of subsequent observers had to reconcile and fill up. For long years Copernicus had brooded over the great thoughts which his careful observation had compelled. We can imagine the touching scene in the little town when his friend Osiander brought the first copy of the precious volume hot from the press, a well enough printed book. Already on his deathbed, stricken with a long illness, the old man must have had doubts how his work would be received, though years before Pope Clement VII had sent him encouraging words. Fortunately death saved him from the "rending" which is the portion of so many innovators and discoverers. His great contemporary reformer, Luther, expressed the view of the day when he said the fool will turn topsy-turvy the whole art of astronomy; but the Bible says that Joshua commanded the Sun to stand still, not the Earth. The scholarly Melanchthon, himself an astronomer, thought the book so godless that he recommended its suppression (Dannemann, Grundriss). The church was too much involved in the Ptolemaic system to accept any change and it was not until 1822 that the works of Copernicus were removed from the Index.

VESALIUS

THE same year, 1542, saw a very different picture in the far-famed city of Padua, "nursery of the arts." The central figure was a man not yet in the prime of life, and justly full of its pride, as you may see from his portrait. Like Aristotle and Hippocrates cradled and nurtured in an AEsculapian family, Vesalius was from his childhood a student of nature, and was now a wandering scholar, far from his Belgian home. But in Italy he had found what neither Louvain nor Paris could give, freedom in his studies and golden opportunities for research in anatomy. What an impression he must have made on the student body at Padua may be judged from the fact that shortly after his graduation in December, 1537, at the age of twenty-four, he was elected to the chair of anatomy and surgery. Two things favored him—an insatiate desire to see and handle for himself the parts of the human frame, and an opportunity, such as had never before been offered to the teacher, to obtain material for the study of human anatomy. Learned with all the learning of the Grecians and of the Arabians, Vesalius grasped, as no modern before him had done, the cardinal fact that to know the human machine and its working, it is necessary first to know its parts—its fabric.

To appreciate the work of this great man we must go back in a brief review of the growth of the study of anatomy.

Among the Greeks only the Alexandrians knew human anatomy. What their knowledge was we know at second hand, but the evidence is plain that they knew a great deal. Galen's anatomy was first-class and was based on the Alexandrians and on his studies of the ape and the pig. We have already noted how much superior was his osteology to that of Mundinus. Between the Alexandrians and the early days of the School of Salernum we have no record of systematic dissections of the human body. It is even doubtful if these were permitted at Salernum. Neuburger states that the instructions of Frederick II as to dissections were merely nominal.

How atrocious was the anatomy of the early Middle Ages may be gathered from the cuts in the works of Henri de Mondeville. In the Bodleian Library is a remarkable Latin anatomical treatise of the late thirteenth century, of English provenance, one illustration from which will suffice to show the ignorance of the author. Mundinus of Bologna, one of the first men in the Middle Ages to study anatomy from the subject, was under the strong domination of the Arabians, from whom he appears to have received a very imperfect Galenic anatomy. From this date we meet with occasional dissections at various schools, but we have seen that in the elaborate curriculum of the University of Padua in the middle of the fifteenth century there was no provision for the study of the subject. Even well into the sixteenth century dissections were not common, and the old practice was followed of holding a professorial discourse, while the butcher, or barber surgeon, opened the cavities of the body. A member of a famous Basel family of physicians, Felix Plater, has left us in his autobiography[19] details of the dissections he witnessed at Montpellier between November 14, 1552, and January 10, 1557, only eleven in number. How difficult it was at that time to get subjects is shown by the risks they ran in "body-snatching" expeditions, of which he records three.

(19) There is no work from which we can get a better idea of the life of the sixteenth-century medical student and of the style of education and of the degree ceremonies, etc. Cumston has given an excellent summary of it (Johns Hopkins Hospital Bulletin, 1912, XXIII, 105-113).

And now came the real maker of modern anatomy. Andreas Vesalius had a good start in life. Of a family long associated with the profession, his father occupied the position of apothecary to Charles V, whom he accompanied on his journeys and campaigns. Trained at Louvain, he had, from his earliest youth, an ardent desire to dissect, and cut up mice and rats, and even cats and dogs. To Paris, the strong school of the period, he went in 1533, and studied under two men of great renown, Jacob Sylvius and Guinterius. Both were strong Galenists and regarded the Master as an infallible authority. He had as a fellow prosector, under the latter, the unfortunate Servetus. The story of his troubles and trials in getting bones and subjects you may read in Roth's "Life."[20] Many interesting biographical details are also to be found in his own writings. He returned for a time to Louvain, and here he published his first book, a commentary on the "Almansor" of Rhazes, in 1537.

(20) M. Roth: Andreas Vesalius Bruxellensis, Berlin, 1892. An excellent account of Vesalius and his contemporaries is given by James Moores Ball in his superbly printed Andreas Vesalius, the Reformer of Anatomy, St. Louis, 1910.

Finding it difficult, either in Paris or Louvain, to pursue his anatomical studies, he decided to go to Italy where, at Venice and Padua, the opportunities were greater. At Venice, he attended the practice of a hospital (now a barracks) which was in charge of the Theatiner Order. I show you a photograph of the building taken last year. And here a strange destiny brought two men together. In 1537, another pilgrim was working in Venice waiting to be joined by his six disciples. After long years of probation, Ignatius Loyola was ready to start on the conquest of a very different world. Devoted to the sick and to the poor, he attached himself to the Theatiner Order, and in the wards of the hospital and the quadrangle, the fiery, dark-eyed, little Basque must frequently have come into contact with the sturdy young Belgian, busy with his clinical studies and his anatomy. Both were to achieve phenomenal success—the one in a few years to revolutionize anatomy, the other within twenty years to be the controller of universities, the counsellor of kings, and the founder of the most famous order in the Roman Catholic Church. It was in this hospital that Vesalius made observations on the China-root, on which he published a monograph in 1546. The Paduan School was close to Venice and associated with it, so that the young student had probably many opportunities of going to and fro. On the sixth of December, 1537, before he had reached his twenty-fourth year and shortly after taking his degree, he was elected to the chair of surgery and anatomy at Padua.

The task Vesalius set himself to accomplish was to give an accurate description of all the parts of the human body, with proper illustrations. He must have had abundant material, more, probably, than any teacher before him had ever had at his disposal. We do not know where he conducted his dissections, as the old amphitheatre has disappeared, but it must have been very different from the tiny one put up by his successor, Fabricius, in 1594. Possibly it was only a temporary building, for he says in the second edition of the "Fabrica" that he had a splendid lecture theatre which accommodated more than five hundred spectators (p. 681).

With Vesalius disappeared the old didactic method of teaching anatomy. He did his own dissections, made his own preparations, and, when human subjects were scarce, employed dogs, pigs or cats, and occasionally a monkey. For five years he taught and worked at Padua. He is known to have given public demonstrations in Bologna and elsewhere. In the 'China-root" he remarks that he once taught in three universities in one year. The first fruit of his work is of great importance in connection with the evolution of his knowledge. In 1538, he published six anatomical tables issued apparently in single leaves. Of the famous "Tabulae Anatomicae" only two copies are known, one in the San Marco Library, Venice, and the other in the possession of Sir John Stirling-Maxwell, whose father had it reproduced in facsimile (thirty copies only) in 1874. Some of the figures were drawn by Vesalius himself, and some are from the pencil of his friend and countryman, Stephan van Calcar. Those plates were extensively pirated. About this time he also edited for the Giunti some of the anatomical works of Galen. (21)

(21) De anatomicis administrationibus, De venarum arterinrumque
    dissectione, included in the various Juntine editions of Galen.

We know very little of his private life at Padua. His most important colleague in the faculty was the famous Montanus, professor of medicine. Among his students and associates was the Englishman Caius, who lived in the same house with him. When the output is considered, he cannot have had much spare time at Padua.

He did not create human anatomy—that had been done by the Alexandrians—but he studied it in so orderly and thorough a manner that for the first time in history it could be presented in a way that explained the entire structure of the human body. Early in 1542 the MS. was ready: the drawings had been made with infinite care, the blocks for the figures had been cut, and in September, he wrote to Oporinus urging that the greatest pains should be taken with the book, that the paper should be strong and of equal thickness, the workmen chosen for their skill, and that every detail of the pictures must be distinctly visible. He writes with the confidence of a man who realized the significance of the work he had done. It is difficult to speak in terms of moderation of the "Fabrica." To appreciate its relative value one must compare it with the other anatomical works of the period, and for this purpose I put before you two figures from a text-book on the subject that was available for students during the first half of the sixteenth century. In the figures and text of the "Fabrica" we have anatomy as we know it; and let us be honest and say, too, largely as Galen knew it. Time will not allow me to go into the question of the relations of these two great anatomists, but we must remember that at this period Galen ruled supreme, and was regarded in the schools as infallible. And now, after five years of incessant labor, Vesalius was prepared to leave his much loved Padua and his devoted students. He had accomplished an extraordinary work. He knew, I feel sure, what he had done. He knew that the MSS. contained something that the world had not seen since the great Pergamenian sent the rolls of his "Manual of Anatomy" among his friends. Too precious to entrust to any printer but the best—and the best in the middle of the sixteenth century was Transalpine—he was preparing to go north with the precious burden. We can picture the youthful teacher—he was but twenty-eight—among students in a university which they themselves controlled—some of them perhaps the very men who five years before had elected him—at the last meeting with his class, perhaps giving a final demonstration of the woodcuts, which were of an accuracy and beauty never seen before by students' eyes, and reading his introduction. There would be sad hearts at the parting, for never had anyone taught anatomy as he had taught it—no one had ever known anatomy as he knew it. But the strong, confident look was on his face and with the courage of youth and sure of the future, he would picture a happy return to attack new and untried problems. Little did he dream that his happy days as student and teacher were finished, that his work as an anatomist was over, that the most brilliant and epoch-making part of his career as a professor was a thing of the past. A year or more was spent at Basel with his friend Oporinus supervising the printing of the great work, which appeared in 1543 with the title "De Humani Corporis Fabrica." The worth of a book, as of a man, must be judged by results, and, so judged, the "Fabrica" is one of the great books of the world, and would come in any century of volumes which embraced the richest harvest of the human mind. In medicine, it represents the full flower of the Renaissance. As a book it is a sumptuous tome a worthy setting of his jewel—paper, type and illustration to match, as you may see for yourselves in this folio—the chef d'oeuvre of any medical library.

In every section, Vesalius enlarged and corrected the work of Galen. Into the details we need not enter: they are all given in Roth's monograph, and it is a chapter of ancient history not specially illuminating.

Never did a great piece of literary work have a better setting. Vesalius must have had a keen appreciation of the artistic side of the art of printing, and he must also have realized the fact that the masters of the art had by this time moved north of the Alps.

While superintending the printing of the precious work in the winter of 1542-1543 in Basel, Vesalius prepared for the medical school a skeleton from the body of an executed man, which is probably the earliest preparation of the kind in Europe. How little anatomy had been studied at the period may be judged from that fact that there had been no dissection at Basel since 1531.(22) The specimen is now in the Vesalianum, Basel, of which I show you a picture taken by Dr. Harvey Cushing. From the typographical standpoint no more superb volume on anatomy has been issued from any press, except indeed the second edition, issued in 1555. The paper is, as Vesalius directed, strong and good, but it is not, as he asked, always of equal thickness; as a rule it is thick and heavy, but there are copies on a good paper of a much lighter quality. The illustrations drawn by his friend and fellow countryman, van Calcar, are very much in advance of anything previously seen, except those of Leonardo. The title-page, one of the most celebrated pictures in the history of medicine, shows Vesalius in a large amphitheatre (an imaginary one of the artist, I am afraid) dissecting a female subject. He is demonstrating the abdomen to a group of students about the table, but standing in the auditorium are elderly citizens and even women. One student is reading from an open book. There is a monkey on one side of the picture and a dog on the other. Above the picture on a shield are the three weasels, the arms of Vesal. The reproduction which I show you here is from the "Epitome"—a smaller work issued before (?) the "Fabrica," with rather larger plates, two of which represent nude human bodies and are not reproduced in the great work. The freshest and most beautiful copy is the one on vellum which formerly belonged to Dr. Mead, now in the British Museum, and from it this picture was taken. One of the most interesting features of the book are the full-page illustrations of the anatomy of the arteries, veins and nerves. They had not in those days the art of making corrosion preparations, but they could in some way dissect to their finest ramifications the arteries, veins and nerves, which were then spread on boards and dried. Several such preparations are now at the College of Physicians in London, brought from Padua by Harvey. The plates of the muscles are remarkably good, more correct, though not better perhaps, on the whole, than some of Leonardo's.

(22) The next, in 1559, is recorded by Plater in his
autobiography, who gave a public dissection during three days in
the Church of St. Elizabeth.

Vesalius had no idea of a general circulation. Though he had escaped from the domination of the great Pergamenian in anatomy, he was still his follower in physiology. The two figures annexed, taken from one of the two existing copies of the "Tabulae Anatomica," are unique in anatomical illustration, and are of special value as illustrating the notion of the vascular system that prevailed until Harvey's day. I have already called your attention to Galen's view of the two separate systems, one containing the coarse, venous blood for the general nutrition of the body, the other the arterial, full of a thinner, warmer blood with which were distributed the vital spirits and the vital heat. The veins had their origin in the liver; the superior vena cava communicated with the right heart, and, as Galen taught, some blood was distributed to the lungs; but the two systems were closed, though Galen believed there was a communication at the periphery between the arteries and veins. Vesalius accepted Galen's view that there is some communication between the venous and arterial systems through pores in the septum of the ventricles, though he had his doubts, and in the second edition of his book (1555) says that inspite of the authority of the Prince of Physicians he cannot see how the smallest quantity of blood could be transmitted through so dense a muscular septum. Two years before this (1553),(*) his old fellow student, Michael Servetus, had in his "Christianismi Restitutio" annatomical touch with one another!

(*) See the Servetus Notes in the Osler Anniversary Volumes, New
York, 1919, Vol. II.—Ed.

The publication of the "Fabrica" shook the medical world to its foundations. Galen ruled supreme in the schools: to doubt him in the least particular roused the same kind of feeling as did doubts on the verbal inspiration of the Scriptures fifty years ago! His old teachers in Paris were up in arms: Sylvius, nostrae aetatis medicorum decus, as Vesalius calls him, wrote furious letters, and later spoke of him as a madman (vaesanus). The younger men were with him and he had many friends, but he had aroused a roaring tide of detraction against which he protested a few years later in his work on the "China-root," which is full of details about the "Fabrica." In a fit of temper he threw his notes on Galen and other MSS. in the fire. No sadder page exists in medical writings than the one in which Vesalius tells of the burning of his books and MSS. It is here reproduced and translated.(23) His life for a couple of years is not easy to follow, but we know that in 1546 he took service with Charles V as his body physician, and the greatest anatomist of his age was lost in the wanderings of court and campaigns. He became an active practitioner, a distinguished surgeon, much consulted by his colleagues, and there are references to many of his cases, the most important of which are to internal aneurysms, which he was one of the first to recognize. In 1555 he brought out the second edition of the "Fabrica," an even more sumptuous volume than the first.

(23) Epistle on China-root, 1546, p. 196. Vesalius may be quoted in explanation—in palliation:

"All these impediments I made light of; for I was too young to seek gain by my art, and I was sustained by my eager desire to learn and to promote the studies in which I shared. I say nothing of my diligence in anatomizing—those who attended my lectures in Italy know how I spent three whole weeks over a single public dissection. But consider that in one year I once taught in three different universities. If I had put off the task of writing till this time; if I were now just beginning to digest my materials; students would not have had the use of my anatomical labours, which posterity may or may not judge superior to the rechauffes formerly in use, whether of Mesua, of Gatinaria, of some Stephanus or other on the differences, causes and symptoms of diseases, or, lastly, of a part of Servitor's pharmacopoeia. As to my notes, which had grown into a huge volume, they were all destroyed by me; and on the same day there similarly perished the whole of my paraphrase on the ten books of Rhazes to King Almansor, which had been composed by me with far more care than the one which is prefaced to the ninth book. With these also went the books of some author or other on the formulae and preparation of medicines, to which I had added much matter of my own which I judged to be not without utility; and the same fate overtook all the books of Galen which I had used in learning anatomy, and which I had liberally disfigured in the usual fashion. I was on the point of leaving Italy and going to Court; those physicians you know of had made to the Emperor and to the nobles a most unfavourable report of my books and of all that is published nowadays for the promotion of study; I therefore burnt all these works that I have mentioned, thinking at the same time that it would be an easy matter to abstain from writing for the future. I must show that I have since repented more than once of my impatience, and regretted that I did not take the advice of the friends who were then with me."

There is no such pathetic tragedy in the history of our profession. Before the age of thirty Vesalius had effected a revolution in anatomy; he became the valued physician of the greatest court of Europe; but call no man happy till he is dead! A mystery surrounds his last days. The story is that he had obtained permission to perform a post-mortem examination on the body of a young Spanish nobleman, whom he had attended. When the body was opened, the spectators to their horror saw the heart beating, and there were signs of life! Accused, so it is said, by the Inquisition of murder and also of general impiety he only escaped through the intervention of the King, with the condition that he make a pilgrimage to the Holy Land. In carrying this out in 1564 he was wrecked on the island of Zante, where he died of a fever or of exhaustion, in the fiftieth year of his age.

To the North American Review, November, 1902, Edith Wharton contributed a poem on "Vesalius in Zante," in which she pictures his life, so full of accomplishment, so full of regrets—regrets accentuated by the receipt of an anatomical treatise by Fallopius, the successor to the chair in Padua! She makes him say:

There are two ways of spreading light; to be
The candle or the mirror that reflects it.
I let my wick burn out—there yet remains
To spread an answering surface to the flame
That others kindle.

But between Mundinus and Vesalius, anatomy had been studied by a group of men to whom I must, in passing, pay a tribute. The great artists Raphael, Michael Angelo and Albrecht Durer were keen students of the human form. There is an anatomical sketch by Michael Angelo in the Ashmolean Museum, Oxford, which I here reproduce. (*) Durer's famous work on "Human Proportion," published in 1528, contains excellent figures, but no sketches of dissections. But greater than any of these, and antedating them, is Leonardo da Vinci, the one universal genius in whom the new spirit was incarnate—the Moses who alone among his contemporaries saw the promised land. How far Leonardo was indebted to his friend and fellow student, della Torre, at Pavia we do not know, nor does it matter in face of the indubitable fact that in the many anatomical sketches from his hand we have the first accurate representation of the structure of the body. Glance at the three figures of the spine which I have had photographed side by side, one from Leonardo, one from Vesalius and the other from Vandyke Carter, who did the drawings in Gray's "Anatomy" (1st ed., 1856). They are all of the same type, scientific, anatomical drawings, and that of Leonardo was done fifty years before Vesalius! Compare, too, this figure of the bones of the foot with a similar one from Vesalius.(24) Insatiate in experiment, intellectually as greedy as Aristotle, painter, poet, sculptor, engineer, architect, mathematician, chemist, botanist, aeronaut, musician and withal a dreamer and mystic, full accomplishment in any one department was not for him! A passionate desire for a mastery of nature's secrets made him a fierce thing, replete with too much rage But for us a record remains—Leonardo was the first of modern anatomists, and fifty years later, into the breach he made, Vesalius entered.(25)

(*) This plate was lacking among the author's illustrations, but the Keeper of the Ashmolean Museum remembers his repeatedly showing special interest in the sketch reproduced in John Addington Symonds's Life of Michelangelo, London, 1893, Vol. I, p. 44, and in Charles Singer's Studies in the History and Method of Science, Oxford, 1917, Vol. I, p. 97, representing Michael Angelo and a friend dissecting the body of a man, by the light of a candle fixed in the body itself.—Ed.

(24) He was the first to make and represent anatomical cross sections. See Leonardo: Quaderni d'Anatomia, Jacob Dybwad, Kristiania, 1911-1916, Vol. V.

(25) See Knox: Great Artists and Great Anatomists, London, 1862, and Mathias Duval in Les Manuserits de Leonard de Vince: De l'Anatomie, Feuillets A, Edouard Rouveyre, Paris, 1898. For a good account of Leonardo da Vinci see Merejkovsky's novel, The Forerunner, London, 1902, also New York, Putnam.

HARVEY

LET us return to Padua about the year 1600. Vesalius, who made the school the most famous anatomical centre in Europe, was succeeded by Fallopius, one of the best-known names in anatomy, at whose death an unsuccessful attempt was made to get Vesalius back. He was succeeded in 1565 by a remarkable man, Fabricius (who usually bears the added name of Aquapendente, from the town of his birth), a worthy follower of Vesalius. In 1594, in the thirtieth year of his professoriate, he built at his own expense a new anatomical amphitheatre, which still exists in the university buildings. It is a small, high-pitched room with six standing-rows for auditors rising abruptly one above the other.

The arena is not much more than large enough for the dissecting table which, by a lift, could be brought up from a preparing room below. The study of anatomy at Padua must have declined since the days of Vesalius if this tiny amphitheatre held all its students; none the less, it is probably the oldest existing anatomical lecture room, and for us it has a very special significance.

Early in his anatomical studies Fabricius had demonstrated the valves in the veins. I show you here two figures, the first, as far as I know, in which these structures are depicted. It does not concern us who first discovered them; they had doubtless been seen before, but Fabricius first recognized them as general structures in the venous system, and he called them little doors—"ostiola."

The quadrangle of the university building at Padua is surrounded by beautiful arcades, the walls and ceilings of which are everywhere covered with the stemmata, or shields, of former students, many of them brilliantly painted. Standing in the arcade on the side of the "quad" opposite the entrance, if one looks on the ceiling immediately above the capital of the second column to the left there is seen the stemma which appears as tailpiece to this chapter, put up by a young Englishman, William Harvey, who had been a student at Padua for four years. He belonged to the "Natio Anglica," of which he was Conciliarius, and took his degree in 1602. Doubtless he had repeatedly seen Fabricius demonstrate the valves of the veins, and he may indeed, as a senior student, have helped in making the very dissections from which the drawings were taken for Fabricius' work, "De Venarum Osteolis," 1603. If one may judge from the character of the teacher's work the sort of instruction the student receives, Harvey must have had splendid training in anatomy. While he was at Padua, the great work of Fabricius, "De Visione, Voce et Auditu" (1600) was published, then the "Tractatus de Oculo Visusque Organo" (1601), and in the last year of his residence Fabricius must have been busy with his studies on the valves of the veins and with his embryology,

which appeared in 1604. Late in life, Harvey told Boyle that it was the position of the valves of the veins that induced him to think of a circulation.

Harvey returned to England trained by the best anatomist of his day. In London, he became attached to the College of Physicans, and taking his degree at Cambridge, he began the practice of medicine. He was elected a fellow of the college in 1607 and physician to St. Bartholomew's Hospital in 1609. In 1615 he was appointed Lumleian lecturer to the College of Physicians, and his duties were to hold certain "public anatomies," as they were called, or lectures. We know little or nothing of what Harvey had been doing other than his routine work in the care of the patients at St. Bartholomew's. It was not until April, 1616, that his lectures began. Chance has preserved to us the notes of this first course; the MS. is now in the British Museum and was published in facsimile by the college in 1886.(26)

(26) William Harvey: Prelectiones Anatomiae Universalis, London, J. & A. Churchill, 1886.

The second day lecture, April 17, was concerned with a description of the organs of the thorax, and after a discussion on the structure and action of the heart come the lines:

W. H. constat per fabricam cordis sanguinem
    per pulmones in Aortam perpetuo transferri, as by two clacks of a water bellows to rayse water
    constat per ligaturam transitum sanguinis
    ab arteriis ad venas
    unde perpetuum sanguinis motum in circulo fieri pulsu cordis.

The illustration will give one an idea of the extraordinarily crabbed hand in which the notes are written, but it is worth while to see the original, for here is the first occasion upon which is laid down in clear and unequivocal words that the blood CIRCULATES. The lecture gave evidence of a skilled anatomist, well versed in the literature from Aristotle to Fabricius. In the MS. of the thorax, or, as he calls it, the "parlour" lecture, there are about a hundred references to some twenty authors. The remarkable thing is that although those lectures were repeated year by year, we have no evidence that they made any impression upon Harvey's contemporaries, so far, at least, as to excite discussions that led to publication. It was not until twelve years later, 1628, that Harvey published in Frankfurt a small quarto volume of seventy-four pages,(27) "De Motu Cordis." In comparison with the sumptuous "Fabrica" of Vesalius this is a trifling booklet; but if not its equal in bulk or typographical beauty (it is in fact very poorly printed), it is its counterpart in physiology, and did for that science what Vesalius had done for anatomy, though not in the same way. The experimental spirit was abroad in the land, and as a student at Padua, Harvey must have had many opportunities of learning the technique of vivisection; but no one before his day had attempted an elaborate piece of experimental work deliberately planned to solve a problem relating to the most important single function of the body. Herein lies the special merit of his work, from every page of which there breathes the modern spirit. To him, as to Vesalius before him, the current views of the movements of the blood were unsatisfactory, more particularly the movements of the heart and arteries, which were regarded as an active expansion by which they were filled with blood, like bellows with air. The question of the transmission of blood through the thick septum and the transference of air and blood from the lungs to the heart were secrets which he was desirous of searching out by means of experiment.

(27) Harvey: Exercitatio Anatomica de Motu Cordis et Sanguinis
in Animalibus, Francofurti, 1628.

One or two special points in the work may be referred to as illustrating his method. He undertook first the movements of the heart, a task so truly arduous and so full of difficulties that he was almost tempted to think with Fracastorius that "the movement of the heart was only to be comprehended by God." But after many difficulties he made the following statements: first, that the heart is erected and raises itself up into an apex, and at this time strikes against the breast and the pulse is felt externally; secondly, that it is contracted every-way, but more so at the sides; and thirdly, that grasped in the hand it was felt to become harder at the time of its motion; from all of which actions Harvey drew the very natural conclusion that the activity of the heart consisted in a contraction of its fibres by which it expelled the blood from the ventricles. These were the first four fundamental facts which really opened the way for the discovery of the circulation, as it did away with the belief that the heart in its motion attracts blood into the ventricles, stating on the contrary that by its contraction it expelled the blood and only received it during its period of repose or relaxation. Then he proceeded to study the action of the arteries and showed that their period of diastole, or expansion, corresponded with the systole, or contraction, of the heart, and that the arterial pulse follows the force, frequency and rhythm of the ventricle and is, in fact, dependent upon it. Here was another new fact: that the pulsation in the arteries was nothing else than the impulse of the blood within them. Chapter IV, in which he describes the movements of the auricles and ventricles, is a model of accurate description, to which little has since been added. It is interesting to note that he mentions what is probably auricular fibrillation. He says: "After the heart had ceased pulsating an undulation or palpitation remained in the blood itself which was contained in the right auricle, this being observed so long as it was imbued with heat and spirit.' He recognized too the importance of the auricles as the first to move and the last to die. The accuracy and vividness of Harvey's description of the motion of the heart have been appreciated by generations of physiologists. Having grasped this first essential fact, that the heart was an organ for the propulsion of blood, he takes up in Chapters VI and VII the question of the conveyance of the blood from the right side of the heart to the left. Galen had already insisted that some blood passed from the right ventricle to the lungs—enough for their nutrition; but Harvey points out, with Colombo, that from the arrangement of the valves there could be no other view than that with each impulse of the heart blood passes from the right ventricle to the lungs and so to the left side of the heart. How it passed through the lungs was a problem: probably by a continuous transudation. In Chapters VIII and IX he deals with the amount of blood passing through the heart from the veins to the arteries. Let me quote here what he says, as it is of cardinal import:

"But what remains to be said upon the quantity and source of the blood which thus passes, is of a character so novel and unheard of that I not only fear injury to myself from the envy of a few, but I tremble lest I have mankind at large for my enemies, so much doth wont and custom become a second nature. Doctrine once sown strikes deeply its root, and respect for antiquity influences all men. Still the die is cast, and my trust is in my love of truth, and the candour of cultivated minds."(28) Then he goes on to say:

(28) William Harvey: Exercitatio Anatomica de Motu Cordis et
Sanguinis in Animalibus,
Francofurti, 1628, G. Moreton's
facsimile reprint and translation,
Canterbury, 1894, p. 48.

"I began to think whether there might not be A MOVEMENT, AS IT WERE, IN A CIRCLE. Now this I afterwards found to be true; and I finally saw that the blood, forced by the action of the left ventricle into the arteries, was distributed to the body at large, and its several parts, in the same manner as it is sent through the lungs, impelled by the right ventricle into the pulmonary artery, and that it then passed through the veins and along the vena cava, and so round to the left ventricle in the manner already indicated."(29)

(29) Ibid. p. 49.

The experiments dealing with the transmission of blood in the veins are very accurate, and he uses the old experiment that Fabricius had employed to show the valves, to demonstrate that the blood in the veins flows towards the heart. For the first time a proper explanation of the action of the valves is given. Harvey had no appreciation of how the arteries and veins communicated with each other. Galen, you may remember, recognized that there were anastomoses, but Harvey preferred the idea of filtration.

The "De Motu Cordis" constitutes a unique piece of work in the history of medicine. Nothing of the same type had appeared before. It is a thoroughly sensible, scientific study of a definite problem, the solution of which was arrived at through the combination of accurate observation and ingenious experiment. Much misunderstanding has arisen in connection with Harvey's discovery of the circulation of the blood. He did not discover that the blood moved,—that was known to Aristotle and to Galen, from both of whom I have given quotations which indicate clearly that they knew of its movement,—but at the time of Harvey not a single anatomist had escaped from the domination of Galen's views. Both Servetus and Colombo knew of the pulmonary circulation, which was described by the former in very accurate terms. Cesalpinus, a great name in anatomy and botany, for whom is claimed the discovery of the circulation, only expressed the accepted doctrines in the following oft-quoted phrase:

"We will now consider how the attraction of aliment and the process of nutrition takes place in plants; for in animals we see the aliment brought through the veins to the heart, as to a laboratory of innate heat, and, after receiving there its final perfection, distributed through the arteries to the body at large, by the agency of the spirits produced from this same aliment in the heart."(30) There is nothing in this but Galen's view, and Cesalpinus believed, as did all his contemporaries, that the blood was distributed through the body by the vena cava and its branches for the nourishment of all its parts.(*) To those who have any doubts as to Harvey's position in this matter I would recommend the reading of the "De Motu Cordis" itself, then the various passages relating to the circulation from Aristotle to Vesalius. Many of these can be found in the admirable works of Dalton, Flourens, Richet and Curtis.(31) In my Harveian Oration for 1906(32) I have dealt specially with the reception of the new views, and have shown how long it was before the reverence for Galen allowed of their acceptance. The University of Paris opposed the circulation of the blood for more than half a century after the appearance of the "De Motu Cordis."

(30) De Plantis, Lib I, cap. 2.

(*) Cesalpinus has also a definite statement of the circlewise
process.—Ed.

(31) J. C. Dalton Doctrines of the Circulation, Philadelphia,
1884; Flourens Histoire de la decouverte de la circulation du
sang, 2d ed., Paris, 1857; Charles Richet Harvey, la circulation
du sang, Paris, 1879; John G. Curtis Harvey's views on the use of
Circulation, etc., New York, 1916.

(32) Osler An Alabama Student and Other Biographical Essays,
Oxford, 1908, p. 295.

To summarize—until the seventeenth century there were believed to be two closed systems in the circulation, (1) the natural, containing venous blood, had its origin in the liver from which, as from a fountain, the blood continually ebbed and flowed for the nourishment of the body; (2) the vital, containing another blood and the spirits, ebbed and flowed from the heart, distributing heat and life to all parts. Like a bellows the lungs fanned and cooled this vital blood. Here and there we find glimmering conceptions of a communication between these systems, but practically all teachers believed that the only one of importance was through small pores in the wall separating the two sides of the heart. Observation—merely looking at and thinking about things—had done all that was possible, and further progress had to await the introduction of a new method, viz., experiment. Galen, it is true, had used this means to show that the arteries of the body contained blood and not air. The day had come when men were no longer content with accurate description and with finely spun theories and dreams. It was reserved for the immortal Harvey to put into practice the experimental method by which he demonstrated conclusively that the blood moved in a circle. The "De Motu Cordis" marks the final break of the modern spirit with the old traditions. It took long for men to realize the value of this "inventum mirabile" used so effectively by the Alexandrians—by Galen—indeed, its full value has only been appreciated within the past century. Let me quote a paragraph from my Harveian Oration.(33) "To the age of the hearer, in which men had heard and heard only, had succeeded the age of the eye in which men had seen and had been content only to see. But at last came the age of the hand—the thinking, devising, planning hand, the hand as an instrument of the mind, now re-introduced into the world in a modest little monograph from which we may date the beginning of experimental medicine."

(33) Osler: An Alabama Student, etc., pp. 329-330.

Harvey caught the experimental spirit in Italy, with brain, eye and hand as his only aids, but now an era opened in which medicine was to derive an enormous impetus from the discovery of instruments of precision. "The new period in the development of the natural sciences, which reached its height in the work of such men as Galileo, Gilbert and Kepler, is chiefly characterized by the invention of very important instruments for aiding and intensifying the perceptions of the senses, by means of which was gained a much deeper insight into the phenomena than had hitherto been possible. Such instruments as the earlier ages possessed were little more than primitive hand-made tools. Now we find a considerable number of scientifically made instruments deliberately planned for purposes of special research, and as it were, on the threshold of the period stand two of the most important, the compound microscope and the telescope. The former was invented about 1590 and the latter about 1608."(34) It was a fellow professor of the great genius Galileo who attempted to put into practice the experimental science of his friend. With Sanctorius began the studies of temperature, respiration and the physics of the circulation. The memory of this great investigator has not been helped by the English edition of his "De Statica Medicina," not his best work, with a frontispiece showing the author in his dietetic balance. Full justice has been done to him by Dr. Weir Mitchell in an address as president of the Congress of Physicians and Surgeons, 1891.(35) Sanctorius worked with a pulsilogue devised for him by Galileo, with which he made observations on the pulse. He is said to have been the first to put in use the clinical thermometer. His experiments on insensible perspiration mark him as one of the first modern physiologists.

(34) Dannemann: Die Naturwissenschaften in ihrer
   Entwickelung., Vol. II, p. 7, Leipzig, 1911.

(35) See Transactions Congress Physicians and Surgeons, 1891, New
   Haven, 1892, II, 159-181.

But neither Sanctorius nor Harvey had the immediate influence upon their contemporaries which the novel and stimulating character of their work justified. Harvey's great contemporary, Bacon, although he lost his life in making a cold storage experiment, did not really appreciate the enormous importance of experimental science. He looked very coldly upon Harvey's work. It was a philosopher of another kidney, Rene Descartes, who did more than anyone else to help men to realize the value of the better way which Harvey had pointed out. That the beginning of wisdom was in doubt, not in authority, was a novel doctrine in the world, but Descartes was no armchair philosopher, and his strong advocacy and practice of experimentation had a profound influence in directing men to "la nouvelle méthode." He brought the human body, the earthly machine, as he calls it, into the sphere of mechanics and physics, and he wrote the first text-book of physiology, "De l'Homme." Locke, too, became the spokesman of the new questioning spirit, and before the close of the seventeenth century, experimental research became all the mode. Richard Lower, Hooke and Hales were probably more influenced by Descartes than by Harvey, and they made notable contributions to experimental physiology in England. Borelli, author of the famous work on "The Motion of Animals" (Rome, 1680-1681), brought to the study of the action of muscles a profound knowledge of physics and mathematics and really founded the mechanical, or iatromechanical school. The literature and the language of medicine became that of physics and mechanics: wheels and pulleys, wedges, levers, screws, cords, canals, cisterns, sieves and strainers, with angles, cylinders, celerity, percussion and resistance, were among the words that now came into use in medical literature. Withington quotes a good example in a description by Pitcairne, the Scot who was professor of medicine at Leyden at the end of the seventeenth century. "Life is the circulation of the blood. Health is its free and painless circulation. Disease is an abnormal motion of the blood, either general or local. Like the English school generally, he is far more exclusively mechanical than are the Italians, and will hear nothing of ferments or acids, even in digestion. This, he declares, is a purely mechanical process due to heat and pressure, the wonderful effects of which may be seen in Papin's recently invented 'digester.' That the stomach is fully able to comminute the food may be proved by the following calculation. Borelli estimates the power of the flexors of the thumb at 3720 pounds, their average weight being 122 grains. Now, the average weight of the stomach is eight ounces, therefore it can develop a force of 117,088 pounds, and this may be further assisted by the diaphragm and abdominal muscles the power of which, estimated in the same way, equals 461,219 pounds! Well may Pitcairne add that this force is not inferior to that of any millstone."(36) Paracelsus gave an extraordinary stimulus to the study of chemistry and more than anyone else he put the old alchemy on modern lines. I have already quoted his sane remark that its chief service is in seeking remedies. But there is another side to this question. If, as seems fairly certain, the Basil Valentine whose writings were supposed to have inspired Paracelsus was a hoax and his works were made up in great part from the writings of Paracelsus, then to our medical Luther, and not to the mythical Benedictine monk, must be attributed a great revival in the search for the Philosopher's Stone, for the Elixir of Life, for a universal medicine, for the perpetuum mobile and for an aurum potabile.(37) I reproduce, almost at random, a page from the fifth and last part of the last will and testament of Basil Valentine (London, 1657), from which you may judge the chemical spirit of the time.

(36) Withington: Medical History from the Earliest Times,
   London, 1891, Scientific Press, p. 317

(37) See Professor Stillman on the Basil Valentine hoax, Popular
   Science Monthly, New York, 1919, LXXXI, 591-600.

Out of the mystic doctrines of Paracelsus arose the famous "Brothers of the Rosy Cross." "The brotherhood was possessed of the deepest knowledge and science, the transmutation of metals, the perpetuum mobile and the universal medicine were among their secrets; they were free from sickness and suffering during their lifetime, though subject finally to death."(38)

(38) Ferguson: Bibliotheca Chemica, Vol. II, p. 290. For an account of Fludd and the English Rosicrucians see Craven's Life of Fludd, Kirkwall, 1902.

A school of a more rational kind followed directly upon the work of Paracelsus, in which the first man of any importance was Van Helmont. The Paracelsian Archeus was the presiding spirit in living creatures, and worked through special local ferments, by which the functions of the organs are controlled. Disease of any part represents a strike on the part of the local Archeus, who refuses to work. Though full of fanciful ideas, Van Helmont had the experimental spirit and was the first chemist to discover the diversity of gases. Like his teacher, he was in revolt against the faculty, and he has bitter things to say of physicians. He got into trouble with the Church about the magnetic cure of wounds, as no fewer than twenty-seven propositions incompatible with the Catholic faith were found in his pamphlet (Ferguson). The Philosophus per ignem, Toparcha in Merode, Royenborch, as he is styled in certain of his writings, is not an easy man to tackle. I show the title-page of the "Ortus Medicinae," the collection of his works by his son. As with the pages of Paracelsus, there are many gems to be dug out. The counterblast against bleeding was a useful protest, and to deny in toto its utility in fever required courage—a quality never lacking in the Father of Modern Chemistry, as he has been called.

A man of a very different type, a learned academic, a professor of European renown, was Daniel Sennert of Wittenberg, the first to introduce the systematic teaching of chemistry into the curriculum, and who tried to harmonize the Galenists and Paracelsians. Franciscus Sylvius, a disciple of Van Helmont, established the first chemical laboratory in Europe at Leyden, and to him is due the introduction of modern clinical teaching. In 1664 he writes: "I have led my pupils by the hand to medical practice, using a method unknown at Leyden, or perhaps elsewhere, i.e., taking them daily to visit the sick at the public hospital. There I have put the symptoms of disease before their eyes; have let them hear the complaints of the patients, and have asked them their opinions as to the causes and rational treatment of each case, and the reasons for those opinions. Then I have given my own judgment on every point. Together with me they have seen the happy results of treatment when God has granted to our cares a restoration of health; or they have assisted in examining the body when the patient has paid the inevitable tribute to death."(39)

(39) Withington: Medical History from the Earliest Times, London, 1894, pp. 312-313.

Glauber, Willis, Mayow, Lemery, Agricola and Stahl led up to Robert Boyle, with whom modern chemistry may be said to begin. Even as late as 1716, Lady Mary Wortley Montagu in Vienna found that all had transferred their superstitions from religion to chemistry; "scarcely a man of opulence or fashion that has not an alchemist in his service. " To one scientific man of the period I must refer as the author of the first scientific book published in England. Dryden sings:

Gilbert shall live till load-stones cease to draw
Or British fleets the boundless ocean awe.

And the verse is true, for by the publication in 1600 of the "De Magnete" the science of electricity was founded. William Gilbert was a fine type of the sixteenth-century physician, a Colchester man, educated at St. John's College, Cambridge. Silvanus Thompson says: "He is beyond question rightfully regarded as the Father of Electric Science. He founded the entire subject of Terrestrial Magnetism. He also made notable contributions to Astronomy, being the earliest English expounder of Copernicus. In an age given over to metaphysical obscurities and dogmatic sophistry, he cultivated the method of experiment and of reasoning from observation, with an insight and success which entitles him to be regarded as the father of the inductive method. That method, so often accredited to Bacon, Gilbert was practicing years before him."(40)

(40) Silvanus P. Thompson: Gilbert of Colchester, Father of Electrical Science, London, Chiswick Press, 1903, p. 3.

CHAPTER V — THE RISE AND DEVELOPMENT OF MODERN MEDICINE

THE middle of the seventeenth century saw the profession thus far on its way—certain objective features of disease were known, the art of careful observation had been cultivated, many empirical remedies had been discovered, the coarser structure of man's body had been well worked out, and a good beginning had been made in the knowledge of how the machinery worked—nothing more. What disease really was, where it was, how it was caused, had not even begun to be discussed intelligently.

An empirical discovery of the first importance marks the middle of the century. The story of cinchona is of special interest, as it was the first great specific in disease to be discovered. In 1638, the wife of the Viceroy of Peru, the Countess of Chinchon, lay sick of an intermittent fever in the Palace of Lima. A friend of her husband's, who had become acquainted with the virtues, in fever, of the bark of a certain tree, sent a parcel of it to the Viceroy, and the remedy administered by her physician, Don Juan del Vego, rapidly effected a cure. In 1640, the Countess returned to Spain, bringing with her a supply of quina bark, which thus became known in Europe as "the Countess's Powder" (pulvis Comitissae). A little later, her doctor followed, bringing additional quantities. Later in the century, the Jesuit Fathers sent parcels of the bark to Rome, whence it was distributed to the priests of the community and used for the cure of ague; hence the name of "Jesuits' bark." Its value was early recognized by Sydenham and by Locke. At first there was a great deal of opposition, and the Protestants did not like it because of its introduction by the Jesuits. The famous quack, Robert Talbor, sold the secret of preparing quinquina to Louis XIV in 1679 for two thousand louis d'or, a pension and a title. That the profession was divided in opinion on the subject was probably due to sophistication, or to the importation of other and inert barks. It was well into the eighteenth century before its virtues were universally acknowledged. The tree itself was not described until 1738, and Linnaeus established the genus "Chinchona" in honor of the Countess.(1)

(1) Clements R. Markham:
Peruvian Bark, John Murray, London, 1880; Memoir of the Lady Anna di Osoria, Countess of Chinchona
and Vice-Queen of Peru, 1874.

A step in advance followed the objective study of the changes wrought in the body by disease. To a few of these the anatomists had already called attention. Vesalius, always keen in his description of aberrations from the normal, was one of the first to describe internal aneurysm. The truth is, even the best of men had little or no appreciation of the importance of the study of these changes. Sydenham scoffs at the value of post-mortems.

Again we have to go back to Italy for the beginning of these studies, this time to Florence, in the glorious days of Lorenzo the Magnificent. The pioneer now is not a professor but a general practitioner, Antonio Benivieni, of whom we know very little save that he was a friend of Marsilio Ficino and of Angelo Poliziano, and that he practiced in Florence during the last third of the fifteenth century, dying in 1502. Through associations with the scholars of the day, he had become a student of Greek medicine and he was not only a shrewd and accurate observer of nature but a bold and successful practitioner. He had formed the good habit of making brief notes of his more important cases, and after his death these were found by his brother Jerome and published in 1507.(2) This book has a rare value as the record of the experience of an unusually intelligent practitioner of the period. There are in all 111 observations, most of them commendably brief. The only one of any length deals with the new "Morbus Gallicus," of which, in the short period between its appearance and Benivieni's death, he had seen enough to leave a very accurate description; and it is interesting to note that even in those early days mercury was employed for its cure. The surgical cases are of exceptional interest, and No. 38 refers to a case of angina for which he performed a successful operation. This is supposed to have been a tracheotomy, and if so, it is the first in the fourteen centuries that had elapsed since the days of Antyllus.(3) There are other important cases which show that he was a dexterous and fearless surgeon But the special interest of the work for us is that, for the first time in modern literature, we have reports of post-mortem examinations made specifically with a view to finding out the exact cause of death. Among the 111 cases, there are post-mortem records of cases of gallstones, abscess of the mesentery, thrombosis of the mesenteric veins, several cases of heart disease, senile gangrene and one of cor villosum. From no other book do we get so good an idea of a practitioner's experience at this period; the notes are plain and straightforward, and singularly free from all theoretical and therapeutic vagaries. He gives several remarkable instances of faith healing.

(2) De abditis nonnullis ac mirandis morborum et sanationum
causis. 8th, Florence, Gandhi, 1507.

(3) Possibly it was only a case of angina Ludovici, or
retro-pharyngeal abscess.

To know accurately the anatomical changes that take place in disease is of importance both for diagnosis and for treatment. The man who created the science, who taught us to think anatomically of disease, was Morgagni, whose "De sedibus et causis morborum per anatomen indagatis"(4) is one of the great books in our literature. During the seventeenth century, the practice of making post-mortem examinations had extended greatly, and in the "Sepulchretum anatomicum" of Bonetus (1679), these scattered fragments are collected.(5) But the work of Morgagni is of a different type, for in it are the clinical and anatomical observations of an able physician during a long and active life. The work had an interesting origin. A young friend interested in science and in medicine was fond of discoursing with Morgagni about his preceptors, particularly Valsalva and Albertini, and sometimes the young man inquired about Morgagni's own observations and thoughts. Yielding to a strong wish, Morgagni consented to write his young friend familiar letters describing his experiences. I am sorry that Morgagni does not mention the name of the man to whom we are so much indebted, and who, he states, was so pleased with the letters that he continually solicited him to send more and more "till he drew me on so far as the seventieth; ... when I begged them of him in order to revise their contents; he did not return them, till he had made me solemnly promise, that I would not abridge any part thereof" (Preface).

(4) Venice, 1761.

(5) Boerhaave remarked that if a man wished to deserve or get a
medical degree from ONE medical author let it be this. (James
Atkinson: Medical Bibliography, 1834, 268.)

Born in 1682, Morgagni studied at Bologna under Valsalva and Albertini. In 1711, he was elected professor of medicine at Padua. He published numerous anatomical observations and several smaller works of less importance. The great work which has made his name immortal in the profession, appeared in his eightieth year, and represents the accumulated experience of a long life. Though written in the form of letters, the work is arranged systematically and has an index of exceptional value. From no section does one get a better idea of the character and scope of the work than from that relating to the heart and arteries—affections of the pericardium, diseases of the valves, ulceration, rupture, dilation and hypertrophy and affections of the aorta are very fully described. The section on aneurysm of the aorta remains one of the best ever written. It is not the anatomical observations alone that make the work of unusual value, but the combination of clinical with anatomical records. What could be more correct than this account of angina pectoris—probably the first in the literature? "A lady forty-two years of age, who for a long time, had been a valetudinarian, and within the same period, on using pretty quick exercise of body, she was subject to attacks of violent anguish in the upper part of the chest on the left side, accompanied with a difficulty of breathing, and numbness of the left arm; but these paroxysms soon subsided when she ceased from exertion. In these circumstances, but with cheerfulness of mind, she undertook a journey from Venice, purposing to travel along the continent, when she was seized with a paroxysm, and died on the spot. I examined the body on the following day. The aorta was considerably dilated at its curvature; and, in places, through its whole tract, the inner surface was unequal and ossified. These appearances were propagated into the arteria innominata. The aortic valves were indurated." He remarks, "The delay of blood in the aorta, in the heart, in the pulmonary vessels, and in the vena cava, would occasion the symptoms of which the woman complained during life; namely, the violent uneasiness, the difficulty of breathing, and the numbness of the arm."(6)

(6) Cooke's Morgagni, Vol. 1, pp. 417-418. I cannot too warmly commend to young clinicians the reading of Morgagni. English editions are available—Alexander's three-volume translation of 1769 and Cooke's Abridgement (London, 1822), of which there was an American edition published in Boston in 1824.

Morgagni's life had as much influence as his work. In close correspondence with the leading men of the day, with the young and rising teachers and workers, his methods must have been a great inspiration; and he came just at the right time. The profession was literally ravaged by theories, schools and systems—iatromechanics, iatrochemistry, humoralism, the animism of Stahl, the vitalistic doctrines of Van Helmont and his followers—and into this metaphysical confusion Morgagni came like an old Greek with his clear observation, sensible thinking and ripe scholarship. Sprengel well remarks that "it is hard to say whether one should admire most his rare dexterity and quickness in dissection, his unimpeachable love of truth and justice in his estimation of the work of others, his extensive scholarship and rich classical style or his downright common sense and manly speech."

Upon this solid foundation the morbid anatomy of modern clinical medicine was built. Many of Morgagni's contemporaries did not fully appreciate the change that was in progress, and the value of the new method of correlating the clinical symptoms and the morbid appearances. After all, it was only the extension of the Hippocratic method of careful observation—the study of facts from which reasonable conclusions could be drawn. In every generation there had been men of this type—I dare say many more than we realize—men of the Benivieni character, thoroughly practical, clear-headed physicians. A model of this sort arose in England in the middle of the seventeenth century, Thomas Sydenham (1624-1689), who took men back to Hippocrates, just as Harvey had led them back to Galen. Sydenham broke with authority and went to nature. It is extraordinary how he could have been so emancipated from dogmas and theories of all sorts. He laid down the fundamental proposition, and acted upon it, that "all disease could be described as natural history." To do him justice we must remember, as Dr. John Brown says, "in the midst of what a mass of errors and prejudices, of theories actively mischievous, he was placed, at a time when the mania of hypothesis was at its height, and when the practical part of his art was overrun and stultified by vile and silly nostrums" ("Horae Subsecivae," Vol. I, 4th ed., Edinburgh, 1882, p. 40).

Listen to what he says upon the method of the study of medicine: "In writing therefore, such a natural history of diseases, every merely philosophical hypothesis should be set aside, and the manifest and natural phenomena, however minute, should be noted with the utmost exactness. The usefulness of this procedure cannot be easily overrated, as compared with the subtle inquiries and trifling notions of modern writers, for can there be a shorter, or indeed any other way of coming at the morbific causes, or discovering the curative indications than by a certain perception of the peculiar symptoms? By these steps and helps it was that the father of physic, the great Hippocrates, came to excel, his theory being no more than an exact description or view of nature. He found that nature alone often terminates diseases, and works a cure with a few simple medicines, and often enough with no medicines at all."

Towards the end of the century many great clinical teachers arose, of whom perhaps the most famous was Boerhaave, often spoken of as the Dutch Hippocrates, who inspired a group of distinguished students. I have already referred to the fact that Franciscus Sylvius at Leyden was the first among the moderns to organize systematic clinical teaching. Under Boerhaave, this was so developed that to this Dutch university students flocked from all parts of Europe. After teaching botany and chemistry, Boerhaave succeeded to the chair of physic in 1714. With an unusually wide general training, a profound knowledge of the chemistry of the day and an accurate acquaintance with all aspects of the history of the profession, he had a strongly objective attitude of mind towards disease, following closely the methods of Hippocrates and Sydenham. He adopted no special system, but studied disease as one of the phenomena of nature. His clinical lectures, held bi-weekly, became exceedingly popular and were made attractive not less by the accuracy and care with which the cases were studied than by the freedom from fanciful doctrines and the frank honesty of the man. He was much greater than his published work would indicate, and, as is the case with many teachers of the first rank, his greatest contributions were his pupils. No other teacher of modern times has had such a following. Among his favorite pupils may be mentioned Haller, the physiologist, and van Swieten and de Haen, the founders of the Vienna school.

In Italy, too, there were men who caught the new spirit, and appreciated the value of combining morbid anatomy with clinical medicine. Lancisi, one of the early students of disease of the heart, left an excellent monograph on the subject, and was the first to call special attention to the association of syphilis with cardio-vascular disease. A younger contemporary of his at Rome, Baglivi, was unceasing in his call to the profession to return to Hippocratic methods, to stop reading philosophical theories and to give up what he calls the "fatal itch" to make systems.

The Leyden methods of instruction were carried far and wide throughout Europe; into Edinburgh by John Rutherford, who began to teach at the Royal Infirmary in 1747, and was followed by Whytt and by Cullen; into England by William Saunders of Guy's Hospital. Unfortunately the great majority of clinicians could not get away from the theoretical conceptions of disease, and Cullen's theory of spasm and atony exercised a profound influence on practice, particularly in this country, where it had the warm advocacy of Benjamin Rush. Even more widespread became the theories of a pupil of Cullen's, John Brown, who regarded excitability as the fundamental property of all living creatures: too much of this excitability produced what were known as sthenic maladies, too little, asthenic; on which principles practice was plain enough. Few systems of medicine have ever stirred such bitter controversy, particularly on the Continent, and in Charles Creighton's account of Brown(7) we read that as late as 1802 the University of Gottingen was so convulsed by controversies as to the merits of the Brunonian system that contending factions of students in enormous numbers, not unaided by the professors, met in combat in the streets on two consecutive days and had to be dispersed by a troop of Hanoverian horse.

(7) Dictionary of National Biography, London, 1886, VII, 14-17.

But the man who combined the qualities of Vesalius, Harvey and Morgagni in an extraordinary personality was John Hunter. He was, in the first place, a naturalist to whom pathological processes were only a small part of a stupendous whole, governed by law, which, however, could never be understood until the facts had been accumulated, tabulated and systematized. By his example, by his prodigious industry, and by his suggestive experiments he led men again into the old paths of Aristotle, Galen and Harvey. He made all thinking physicians naturalists, and he lent a dignity to the study of organic life, and reestablished a close union between medicine and the natural sciences. Both in Britain and Greater Britain, he laid the foundation of the great collections and museums, particularly those connected with the medical schools. The Wistar-Horner and the Warren Museums in this country originated with men greatly influenced by Hunter. He was, moreover, the intellectual father of that interesting group of men on this side of the Atlantic who, while practising as physicians, devoted much time and labor to the study of natural history; such men as Benjamin Smith Barton, David Hossack, Jacob Bigelow, Richard Harlan, John D. Godman, Samuel George Morton, John Collins Warren, Samuel L. Mitchill and J. Aitken Meigs. He gave an immense impetus in Great Britain to the study of morbid anatomy, and his nephew, Matthew Baillie, published the first important book on the subject in the English language.

Before the eighteenth century closed practical medicine had made great advance. Smallpox, though not one of the great scourges like plague or cholera, was a prevalent and much dreaded disease, and in civilized countries few reached adult life without an attack. Edward Jenner, a practitioner in Gloucestershire, and the pupil to whom John Hunter gave the famous advice: "Don't think, try!" had noticed that milkmaids who had been infected with cowpox from the udder of the cow were insusceptible to smallpox. I show you here the hand of Sarah Nelmes with cowpox, 1796. A vague notion had prevailed among the dairies from time immemorial that this disease was a preventive of the smallpox. Jenner put the matter to the test of experiment. Let me quote here his own words: "The first experiment was made upon a lad of the name of Phipps, in whose arm a little vaccine virus was inserted, taken from the hand of a young woman who had been accidentally infected by a cow. Notwithstanding the resemblance which the pustule, thus excited on the boy's arm, bore to variolous inoculation, yet as the indisposition attending it was barely perceptible, I could scarcely persuade myself the patient was secure from the Small Pox. However, on his being inoculated some months afterwards, it proved that he was secure."(8) The results of his experiments were published in a famous small quarto volume in 1793.(*) From this date, smallpox has been under control. Thanks to Jenner, not a single person in this audience is pockmarked! A hundred and twenty-five years ago, the faces of more than half of you would have been scarred. We now know the principle upon which protection is secured: an active acquired immunity follows upon an attack of a disease of a similar nature. Smallpox and cowpox are closely allied and the substances formed in the blood by the one are resistant to the virus of the other. I do not see how any reasonable person can oppose vaccination or decry its benefits. I show you the mortality figures(9) of the Prussian Army and of the

German Empire. A comparison with the statistics of the armies of other European countries in which revaccination is not so thoroughly carried out is most convincing of its efficacy.

(8) Edward Jenner: The Origin of the Vaccine Inoculation,
London, 1801.

(*) Reprinted by Camac: Epoch-making Contributions to Medicine, etc., 1909.—Ed.

(9) Jockmann: Pocken und Vaccinationlehre, 1913.

The early years of the century saw the rise of modern clinical medicine in Paris. In the art of observation men had come to a standstill. I doubt very much whether Corvisart in 1800 was any more skilful in recognizing a case of pneumonia than was Aretaeus in the second century A. D. But disease had come to be more systematically studied; special clinics were organized, and teaching became much more thorough. Anyone who wishes to have a picture of the medical schools in Europe in the first few years of the century, should read the account of the travels of Joseph Frank of Vienna.(10) The description of Corvisart is of a pioneer in clinical teaching whose method remains in vogue today in France—the ward visit, followed by a systematic lecture in the amphitheatre. There were still lectures on Hippocrates three times a week, and bleeding was the principal plan of treatment: one morning Frank saw thirty patients, out of one hundred and twelve, bled! Corvisart was the strong clinician of his generation, and his accurate studies on the heart were among the first that had concentrated attention upon a special organ. To him, too, is due the reintroduction of the art of percussion in internal disease discovered by Auenbrugger in 1761.

(10) Joseph Frank: Reise nach Paris (etc.), Wien, 1804-05.

The man who gave the greatest impetus to the study of scientific medicine at this time was Bichat, who pointed out that the pathological changes in disease were not so much in organs as in tissues. His studies laid the foundation of modern histology. He separated the chief constituent elements of the body into various tissues possessing definite physical and vital qualities. "Sensibility and contractability are the fundamental qualities of living matter and of the life of our tissues. Thus Bichat substituted for vital forces 'vital properties,' that is to say, a series of vital forces inherent in the different tissues."(11) His "Anatomic Generale," published in 1802, gave an extraordinary stimulus to the study of the finer processes of disease, and his famous "Recherches sur la Vie et sur la Mort" (1800) dealt a death-blow to old iatromechanical and iatrochemical views. His celebrated definition may be quoted: "La vie est l'ensemble des proprietes vitales qui resistent aux proprietes physiques, ou bien la vie est l'ensemble des fonctions qui resistent a la mort." (Life is the sum of the vital properties that withstand the physical properties, or, life is the sum of the functions that withstand death.) Bichat is another pathetic figure in medical history. His meteoric career ended in his thirty-first year: he died a victim of a post-mortem wound infection. At his death, Corvisart wrote Napoleon: "Bichat has just died at the age of thirty. That battlefield on which he fell is one which demands courage and claims many victims. He has advanced the science of medicine. No one at his age has done so much so well."

(11) E. Boinet: Les doctrines medicules, leur evolution, Paris, 1907, pp. 85-86.

It was a pupil of Corvisart, Rene Theophile Laennec, who laid the foundation of modern clinical medicine. The story of his life is well known. A Breton by birth, he had a hard, up-hill struggle as a young man—a struggle of which we have only recently been made aware by the publication of a charming book by Professor Rouxeau of Nantes—"Laennec avant 1806." Influenced by Corvisart, he began to combine the accurate study of cases in the wards with anatomical investigations in the dead-house. Before Laennec, the examination of a patient had been largely by sense of sight, supplemented by that of touch, as in estimating the degree of fever, or the character of the pulse. Auenbrugger's "Inventum novum" of percussion, recognized by Corvisart, extended the field; but the discovery of auscultation by Laennec, and the publication of his work—"De l'Auscultation Mediate," 1819,—marked an era in the study of medicine. The clinical recognition of individual diseases had made really very little progress; with the stethoscope begins the day of physical diagnosis. The clinical pathology of the heart, lungs and abdomen was revolutionized. Laennec's book is in the category of the eight or ten greatest contributions to the science of medicine.(*) His description of tuberculosis is perhaps the most masterly chapter in clinical medicine. This revolution was effected by a simple extension of the Hippocratic method from the bed to the dead-house, and by correlating the signs and symptoms of a disease with its anatomical appearances.

(*) John Forbes's translation of Auenbrugger and part of his
translation of Lacnnec are reprinted in Camac's Epoch-making
Contributions, etc., 1909.—Ed.

The pupils and successors of Corvisart—Bayle, Andral, Bouillaud, Chomel, Piorry, Bretonneau, Rayer, Cruveilhier and Trousseau—brought a new spirit into the profession. Everywhere the investigation of disease by clinical-pathological methods widened enormously the diagnostic powers of the physician. By this method Richard Bright, in 1836, opened a new chapter on the relation of disease of the kidney to dropsy, and to albuminous urine. It had already been shown by Blackwell and by Wells, the celebrated Charleston (S.C.) physician, in 1811, that the urine contained albumin in many cases of dropsy, but it was not until Bright began a careful investigation of the bodies of patients who had presented these symptoms, that he discovered the association of various forms of disease of the kidney with anasarca and albuminous urine. In no direction was the harvest of this combined study more abundant than in the complicated and confused subject of fever. The work of Louis and of his pupils, W.W. Gerhard and others, revealed the distinction between typhus and typhoid fever, and so cleared up one of the most obscure problems in pathology. By Morgagni's method of "anatomical thinking," Skoda in Vienna, Schonlein in Berlin, Graves and Stokes in Dublin, Marshall Hall, C. J. B. Williams and many others introduced the new and exact methods of the French and created a new clinical medicine. A very strong impetus was given by the researches of Virchow on cellular pathology, which removed the seats of disease from the tissues, as taught by Bichat, to the individual elements, the cells. The introduction of the use of the microscope in clinical work widened greatly our powers of diagnosis, and we obtained thereby a very much clearer conception of the actual processes of disease. In another way, too, medicine was greatly helped by the rise of experimental pathology, which had been introduced by John Hunter, was carried along by Magendie and others, and reached its culmination in the epoch-making researches of Claude Bernard. Not only were valuable studies made on the action of drugs, but also our knowledge of cardiac pathology was revolutionized by the work of Traube, Cohnheim and others. In no direction did the experimental method effect such a revolution as in our knowledge of the functions of the brain. Clinical neurology, which had received a great impetus by the studies of Todd, Romberg, Lockhart Clarke, Duchenne and Weir Mitchell, was completely revolutionized by the experimental work of Hitzig, Fritsch and Ferrier on the localization of functions in the brain. Under Charcot, the school of French neurologists gave great accuracy to the diagnosis of obscure affections of the brain and spinal cord, and the combined results of the new anatomical, physiological and experimental work have rendered clear and definite what was formerly the most obscure and complicated section of internal medicine. The end of the fifth decade of the century is marked by a discovery of supreme importance. Humphry Davy had noted the effects of nitrous oxide. The exhilarating influence of sulphuric ether had been casually studied, and Long of Georgia had made patients inhale the vapor until anaesthetic and had performed operations upon them when in this state; but it was not until October 16, 1846, in the Massachusetts General Hospital, that Morton, in a public operating room, rendered a patient insensible with ether and demonstrated the utility of surgical anaesthesia. The rival claims of priority no longer interest us, but the occasion is one of the most memorable in the history of the race. It is well that our colleagues celebrate Ether Day in Boston—no more precious boon has ever been granted to suffering humanity.(*)

(*) Cf. Osler: Proc. Roy. Soc. Med. , XI, Sect. Hist Med., pp.
65-69, 1918, or, Annals Med. Hist., N.Y., I, 329-332. Cf. also
Morton's publications reprinted in Camac's book cited above.—Ed.

In 1857, a young man, Louis Pasteur, sent to the Lille Scientific Society a paper on "Lactic Acid Fermentation" and in December of the same year presented to the Academy of Sciences in Paris a paper on "Alcoholic Fermentation" in which he concluded that "the deduplication of sugar into alcohol and carbonic acid is correlative to a phenomenon of life." A new era in medicine dates from those two publications. The story of Pasteur's life should be read by every student.(*) It is one of the glories of human literature, and, as a record of achievement and of nobility of character, is almost without an equal.

(*) Osler wrote a preface for the 1911 English edition of the
Life by Vallery-Radot.—Ed.

At the middle of the last century we did not know much more of the actual causes of the great scourges of the race, the plagues, the fevers and the pestilences, than did the Greeks. Here comes Pasteur's great work. Before him Egyptian darkness; with his advent a light that brightens more and more as the years give us ever fuller knowledge. The facts that fevers were catching, that epidemics spread, that infection could remain attached to articles of clothing, etc., all gave support to the view that the actual cause was something alive, a contagium vivum. It was really a very old view, the germs of which may be found in the Fathers, but which was first clearly expressed—so far as I know—by Fracastorius, the Veronese physician, in the sixteenth century, who spoke of the seeds of contagion passing from one person to another;(12) and he first drew a parallel between the processes of contagion and the fermentation of wine. This was more than one hundred years before Kircher, Leeuwenhoek and others began to use the microscope and to see animalcula, etc, in water, and so give a basis for the "infinitely little" view of the nature of disease germs. And it was a study of the processes of fermentation that led Pasteur to the sure ground on which we now stand.

(12) Varro, in De Re Rustica, Bk. I, 12 (circa 40 B.C.), speaks
of minute organisms which the eye cannot see and which enter the
body and cause disease.

Out of these researches arose a famous battle which kept Pasteur hard at work for four or five years—the struggle over spontaneous generation. It was an old warfare, but the microscope had revealed a new world, and the experiments on fermentation had lent great weight to the omne vivum ex ovo doctrine. The famous Italians, Redi and Spallanzani, had led the way in their experiments, and the latter had reached the conclusion that there is no vegetable and no animal that has not its own germ. But heterogenesis became the burning question, and Pouchet in France, and Bastian in England, led the opposition to Pasteur. The many famous experiments carried conviction to the minds of scientific men, and destroyed forever the old belief in spontaneous generation. All along, the analogy between disease and fermentation must have been in Pasteur's mind; and then came the suggestion, "What would be most desirable is to push those studies far enough to prepare the road for a serious research into the origin of various diseases." If the changes in lactic, alcoholic and butyric fermentations are due to minute living organisms, why should not the same tiny creatures make the changes which occur in the body in the putrid and suppurative diseases? With an accurate training as a chemist, having been diverted in his studies upon fermentation into the realm of biology, and nourishing a strong conviction of the identity between putrefactive changes of the body and fermentation, Pasteur was well prepared to undertake investigations which had hitherto been confined to physicians alone.

So impressed was he with the analogy between fermentation and the infectious diseases that, in 1863, he assured the French Emperor of his ambition "to arrive at the knowledge of the causes of putrid and contagious diseases." After a study upon the diseases of wines, which has had most important practical bearings, an opportunity arose which changed the whole course of his career, and profoundly influenced the development of medical science. A disease of the silkworm had, for some years, ruined one of the most important industries in France, and in 1865 the Government asked Pasteur to give up his laboratory work and teaching, and to devote his whole energies to the task of investigating it. The story of the brilliant success which followed years of application to the problem will be read with deep interest by every student of science. It was the first of his victories in the application of the experimental methods of a trained chemist to the problems of biology, and it placed his name high in the group of the most illustrious benefactors of practical industries.

In a series of studies on the diseases of beer, and on the mode of production of vinegar, he became more and more convinced that these studies on fermentation had given him the key to the nature of the infectious diseases. It is a remarkable fact that the distinguished English philosopher of the seventeenth century, the man who more than anyone else of his century appreciated the importance of the experimental method, Robert Boyle, had said that he who could discover the nature of ferments and fermentation, would be more capable than anyone else of explaining the nature of certain diseases.

In 1876 there appeared in Cohn's "Beitrage zur Morphologie der Pflanzen" (II, 277-310), a paper on the "AEtiology of Anthrax" by a German district physician in Wollstein, Robert Koch, which is memorable in our literature as the starting point of a new method of research into the causation of infectious diseases. Koch demonstrated the constant presence of germs in the blood of animals dying from the disease. Years before, those organisms had been seen by Pollender and Davaine, but the epoch-making advance of Koch was to grow those organisms in a pure culture outside the body, and to produce the disease artificially by inoculating animals with the cultures Koch is really our medical Galileo, who, by means of a new technique,—pure cultures and isolated staining,—introduced us to a new world. In 1878, followed his study on the "AEtiology of Wound Infections," in which he was able to demonstrate conclusively the association of microorganisms with the disease. Upon those two memorable researches made by a country doctor rests the modern science of bacteriology.

The next great advance was the discovery by Pasteur of the possibility of so attenuating, or weakening, the poison that an animal inoculated had a slight attack, recovered and was then protected against the disease. More than eighty years had passed since on May 14, 1796, Jenner had vaccinated a child with cowpox and proved that a slight attack of one disease protected the body from a disease of an allied nature. An occasion equally famous in the history of medicine was a day in 1881, when Pasteur determined that a flock of sheep vaccinated with the attenuated virus of anthrax remained well, when every one of the unvaccinated infected from the same material had died. Meanwhile, from Pasteur's researches on fermentation and spontaneous generation, a transformation had been initiated in the practice of surgery, which, it is not too much to say, has proved one of the greatest boons ever conferred upon humanity. It had long been recognized that, now and again, a wound healed without the formation of pus, that is, without suppuration, but both spontaneous and operative wounds were almost invariably associated with that process; and, moreover, they frequently became putrid, as it was then called,— infected, as we should say,—the general system became involved and the patient died of blood poisoning. So common was this, particularly in old, ill-equipped hospitals, that many surgeons feared to operate, and the general mortality in all surgical cases was very high. Believing that it was from outside that the germs came which caused the decomposition of wounds, just as from the atmosphere the sugar solution got the germs which caused the fermentation, a young surgeon in Glasgow, Joseph Lister, applied the principles of Pasteur's experiments to their treatment. From Lister's original paper(*) I quote the following: "Turning now to the question how the atmosphere produces decomposition of organic substances, we find that a flood of light has been thrown upon this most important subject by the philosophic researches of M. Pasteur, who has demonstrated by thoroughly convincing evidence that it is not to its oxygen or to any of its gaseous constituents that the air owes this property, but to minute particles suspended in it, which are the germs of various low forms of life, long since revealed by the microscope, and regarded as merely accidental concomitants of putrescence, but now shown by Pasteur to be its essential cause, resolving the complex organic compounds into substances of simpler chemical constitution, just as the yeast-plant converts sugar into alcohol and carbonic acid." From these beginnings modern surgery took its rise, and the whole subject of wound infection, not only in relation to surgical diseases, but to child-bed fever, forms now one of the most brilliant chapters in the history of preventive medicine.

(*) Lancet, March 16, 1867. (Cf. Camac: Epoch-making
  Contributions, etc., 1909, p. 7.—Ed.
)

With the new technique and experimental methods, the discovery of the specific germs of many of the more important acute infections followed each other with bewildering rapidity: typhoid fever, diphtheria, cholera, tetanus, plague, pneumonia, gonorrhoea and, most important of all, tuberculosis. It is not too much to say that the demonstration by Koch of the "bacillus tuberculosis" (1882) is, in its far-reaching results, one of the most momentous discoveries ever made.

Of almost equal value have been the researches upon the protozoan forms of animal life, as causes of disease. As early as 1873, spirilla were demonstrated in relapsing fever. Laveran proved the association of haematozoa with malaria in 1880. In the same year, Griffith Evans discovered trypanosomes in a disease of horses and cattle in India, and the same type of parasite was found in the sleeping sickness. Amoebae were demonstrated in one form of dysentery, and in other tropical diseases protozoa were discovered, so that we were really prepared for the announcement in 1905, by Schaudinn, of the discovery of a protozoan parasite in syphilis. Just fifty years had passed since Pasteur had sent in his paper on "Lactic Acid Fermentation" to the Lille Scientific Society— half a century in which more had been done to determine the true nature of disease than in all the time that had passed since Hippocrates. Celsus makes the oft-quoted remark that to determine the cause of a disease often leads to the remedy,(*) and it is the possibility of removing the cause that gives such importance to the new researches on disease.

(*) "Et causae quoque estimatio saepe morbum solvit," Celsus, Lib. I, Prefatio.—Ed.

INTERNAL SECRETIONS

ONE of the greatest contributions of the nineteenth century to scientific medicine was the discovery of the internal secretions of organs. The basic work on the subject was done by Claude Bernard, a pupil of the great Magendie, whose saying it is well to remember— "When entering a laboratory one should leave theories in the cloakroom." More than any other man of his generation, Claude Bernard appreciated the importance of experiment in practical medicine. For him the experimental physician was the physician of the future— a view well borne out by the influence his epoch-making work has had on the treatment of disease. His studies on the glycogenic functions of the liver opened the way for the modern fruitful researches on the internal secretions of the various glands. About the same time that Bernard was developing the laboratory side of the problem, Addison, a physician to Guy's Hospital, in 1855, pointed out the relation of a remarkable group of symptoms to disease of the suprarenal glands, small bodies situated above the kidneys, the importance of which had not been previously recognized. With the loss of the function of these glands by disease, the body was deprived of something formed by them which was essential to its proper working. Then, in the last third of the century, came in rapid succession the demonstration of the relations of the pancreas to diabetes, of the vital importance of the thyroid gland and of the pituitary body. Perhaps no more striking illustration of the value of experimental medicine has ever been given than that afforded by the studies upon those glands.

The thyroid body, situated in the neck and the enlargement of which is called goitre, secretes substances which pass into the blood, and which are necessary for the growth of the body in childhood, for the development of the mind and for the nutrition of the tissues of the skin. If, following an infectious disease, a child has wasting of this gland, or if, living in a certain district, it has a large goitre, normal development does not take place, and the child does not grow in mind or body and becomes what is called a cretin. More than this—if in adult life the gland is completely removed, or if it wastes, a somewhat similar condition is produced, and the patient in time loses his mental powers and becomes fat and flabby—myxedematous. It has been shown experimentally in various ways that the necessary elements of the secretion can be furnished by feeding with the gland or its extracts, and that the cretinoid or myxedematous conditions could thus be cured or prevented.

Experimental work has also demonstrated the functions of the suprarenal glands and explained the symptoms of Addison's disease, and chemists have even succeeded in making synthetically the active principle adrenalin.

There is perhaps no more fascinating story in the history of science than that of the discovery of these so-called ductless glands. Part of its special interest is due to the fact that clinicians, surgeons, experimental physiologists, pathologists and chemists have all combined in splendid teamwork to win the victory. No such miracles have ever before been wrought by physicians as those which we see in connection with the internal secretion of the thyroid gland. The myth of bringing the dead back to life has been associated with the names of many great healers since the incident of Empedocles and Pantheia, but nowadays the dead in mind and the deformed in body may be restored by the touch of the magic wand of science. The study of the interaction of these internal secretions, their influence upon development, upon mental process and upon disorders of metabolism is likely to prove in the future of a benefit scarcely less remarkable than that which we have traced in the infectious diseases.

CHEMISTRY

IT is not making too strong a statement to say that the chemistry and chemical physics of the nineteenth century have revolutionized the world. It is difficult to realize that Liebig's famous Giessen laboratory, the first to be opened to students for practical study, was founded in the year 1825. Boyle, Cavendish, Priestley, Lavoisier, Black, Dalton and others had laid a broad foundation, and Young, Frauenhofer, Rumford, Davy, Joule, Faraday, Clerk-Maxwell, Helmholtz and others built upon that and gave us the new physics and made possible our age of electricity. New technique and new methods have given a powerful stimulus to the study of the chemical changes that take place in the body, which, only a few years ago, were matters largely of speculation. "Now," in the words of Professor Lee, "we recognize that, with its living and its non-living substances inextricably intermingled, the body constitutes an intensive chemical laboratory in which there is ever occurring a vast congeries of chemical reactions; both constructive and destructive processes go on; new protoplasm takes the place of old. We can analyze the income of the body and we can analyze its output, and from these data we can learn much concerning the body's chemistry. A great improvement in the method of such work has recently been secured by the device of inclosing the person who is the subject of the experiment in a respiration calorimeter. This is an air-tight chamber, artificially supplied with a constant stream of pure air, and from which the expired air, laden with the products of respiration, is withdrawn for purposes of analysis. The subject may remain in the chamber for days, the composition of all food and all excrete being determined, and all heat that is given off being measured. Favorable conditions are thus established for an exact study of many problems of nutrition. The difficulties increase when we attempt to trace the successive steps in the corporeal pathway of molecule and atom. Yet these secrets of the vital process are also gradually being revealed. When we remember that it is in this very field of nutrition that there exist great popular ignorance and a special proneness to fad and prejudice, we realize how practically helpful are such exact studies of metabolism."(13)

(13) Frederick S. Lee, Ph.D.: Scientific Features of Modern Medicine, New York, 1911. I would like to call attention to this work of Professor Lee's as presenting all the scientific features of modern medicine in a way admirably adapted for anyone, lay or medical, who wishes to get a clear sketch of them.

CHAPTER VI — THE RISE OF PREVENTIVE MEDICINE

THE story so far has been of men and of movements—of men who have, consciously or unconsciously, initiated great movements, and of movements by which, nolens volens, the men of the time were moulded and controlled. Hippocrates, in the tractate on "Ancient Medicine," has a splendid paragraph on the attitude of mind towards the men of the past. My attention was called to it one day in the Roman Forum by Commendatore Boni, who quoted it as one of the great sayings of antiquity. Here it is: "But on that account, I say, we ought not to reject the ancient Art, as if it were not, and had not been properly founded, because it did not attain accuracy in all things, but rather, since it is capable of reaching to the greatest exactitude by reasoning, to receive it and admire its discoveries, made from a state of great ignorance, and as having been well and properly made, and not from chance."(1)

(1) The Works of Hippocrates, Adams, Vol. I, p. 168, London, 1849 (Sydenham Society).

I have tried to tell you what the best of these men in successive ages knew, to show you their point of outlook on the things that interest us. To understand the old writers one must see as they saw, feel as they felt, believe as they believed—and this is hard, indeed impossible! We may get near them by asking the Spirit of the Age in which they lived to enter in and dwell with us, but it does not always come. Literary criticism is not literary history—we have no use here for the former, but to analyze his writings is to get as far as we can behind the doors of a man's mind, to know and appraise his knowledge, not from our standpoint, but from that of his contemporaries, his predecessors and his immediate successors. Each generation has its own problems to face, looks at truth from a special focus and does not see quite the same outlines as any other. For example, men of the present generation grow up under influences very different from those which surrounded my generation in the seventies of the last century, when Virchow and his great contemporaries laid the sure and deep foundations of modern pathology. Which of you now knows the "Cellular Pathology" as we did? To many of you it is a closed book,—to many more Virchow may be thought a spent force. But no, he has only taken his place in a great galaxy. We do not forget the magnitude of his labors, but a new generation has new problems—his message was not for you—but that medicine today runs in larger moulds and turns out finer castings is due to his life and work. It is one of the values of lectures on the history of medicine to keep alive the good influences of great men even after their positive teaching is antiquated. Let no man be so foolish as to think that he has exhausted any subject for his generation. Virchow was not happy when he saw the young men pour into the old bottle of cellular pathology the new wine of bacteriology. Lister could never understand how aseptic surgery arose out of his work. Ehrlich would not recognize his epoch-making views on immunity when this generation has finished with them. I believe it was Hegel who said that progress is a series of negations—the denial today of what was accepted yesterday, the contradiction by each generation of some part at least of the philosophy of the last; but all is not lost, the germ plasm remains, a nucleus of truth to be fertilized by men often ignorant even of the body from which it has come. Knowledge evolves, but in such a way that its possessors are never in sure possession. "It is because science is sure of nothing that it is always advancing" (Duclaux).

History is the biography of the mind of man, and its educational value is in direct proportion to the completeness of our study of the individuals through whom this mind has been manifested. I have tried to take you back to the beginnings of science, and to trace its gradual development, which is conditioned by three laws. In the first place, like a living organism, truth grows, and its gradual evolution may be traced from the tiny germ to the mature product. Never springing, Minerva-like, to full stature at once, truth may suffer all the hazards incident to generation and gestation. Much of history is a record of the mishaps of truths which have struggled to the birth, only to die or else to wither in premature decay. Or the germ may be dormant for centuries, awaiting the fullness of time.

Secondly, all scientific truth is conditioned by the state of knowledge at the time of its announcement. Thus, at the beginning of the seventeenth century, the science of optics and mechanical appliances had not made possible (so far as the human mind was concerned) the existence of blood capillaries and blood corpuscles. Jenner could not have added to his "Inquiry" a study on immunity; Sir William Perkin and the chemists made Koch technique possible; Pasteur gave the conditions that produced Lister; Davy and others furnished the preliminaries necessary for anaesthesia. Everywhere we find this filiation, one event following the other in orderly sequence—"Mind begets mind," as Harvey (De Generatione) says; "opinion is the source of opinion. Democritus with his atoms, and Eudoxus with his chief good which he placed in pleasure, impregnated Epicurus; the four elements of Empedocles, Aristotle; the doctrines of the ancient Thebans, Pythagoras and Plato; geometry, Euclid."(2)

(2) Works of William Harvey, translated by Robert Willis, London, 1847, p. 532.

And, thirdly, to scientific truth alone may the homo mensura principle be applied, since of all mental treasures of the race it alone compels general acquiescence. That this general acquiescence, this aspect of certainty, is not reached per saltum, but is of slow, often of difficult growth,—marked by failures and frailties, but crowned at last with an acceptance accorded to no other product of mental activity,—is illustrated by every important discovery from Copernicus to Darwin.

The difficulty is to get men to the thinking level which compels the application of scientific truths. Protagoras, that "mighty-wise man," as Socrates called him, who was responsible for the aphorism that man is the measure of all things, would have been the first to recognize the folly of this standard for the people at large. But we have gradually reached a stage in which knowledge is translated into action, made helpful for suffering humanity, just as the great discoveries in physics and chemistry have been made useful in the advance of civilization. We have traced medicine through a series of upward steps—a primitive stage, in which it emerged from magic and religion into an empirical art, as seen among the Egyptians and Babylonians; a stage in which the natural character of disease was recognized and the importance of its study as a phenomenon of nature was announced; a stage in which the structure and functions of the human body were worked out; a stage in which the clinical and anatomical features of disease were determined; a stage in which the causes of disorders were profitably studied, and a final stage, into which we have just entered, the application of the knowledge for their prevention. Science has completely changed man's attitude towards disease.

Take a recent concrete illustration. A couple of years ago in Philadelphia and in some other parts of the United States, a very peculiar disease appeared, characterized by a rash upon the skin and moderate fever, and a constitutional disturbance proportionate to the extent and severity of the eruption. The malady first broke out in the members of a crew of a private yacht; then in the crews of other boats, and among persons living in the boarding-houses along the docks. It was the cause of a great deal of suffering and disability.

There were three courses open: to accept the disease as a visitation of God, a chastening affliction sent from above, and to call to aid the spiritual arm of the church. Except the "Peculiar People" few now take this view or adopt this practice. The Christian Scientist would probably deny the existence of the rash and of the fever, refuse to recognize the itching and get himself into harmony with the Infinite. Thirdly, the method of experimental medicine.

First, the conditions were studied under which the individual cases occurred. The only common factor seemed to be certain straw mattresses manufactured by four different firms, all of which obtained the straw from the same source.

The second point was to determine the relation of the straw to the rash. One of the investigators exposed a bare arm and shoulder for an hour between two mattresses. Three people voluntarily slept on the mattresses for one night. Siftings from the straw were applied to the arm, under all of which circumstances the rash quickly developed, showing conclusively the relation of the straw to the disease.

Thirdly, siftings from the straw and mattresses which had been thoroughly disinfected failed to produce the rash.

And fourthly, careful inspection of the siftings of the straw disclosed living parasites, small mites, which when applied to the skin quickly produced the characteristic eruption.

SANITATION

WHEN the thoughtful historian gets far enough away from the nineteenth century to see it as a whole, no single feature will stand out with greater distinctness than the fulfilment of the prophecy of Descartes that we could be freed from an infinity of maladies both of body and mind if we had sufficient knowledge of their causes and of all the remedies with which nature has provided us. Sanitation takes its place among the great modern revolutions—political, social and intellectual. Great Britain deserves the credit for the first practical recognition of the maxim salus populi suprema lex. In the middle and latter part of the century a remarkable group of men, Southwood Smith, Chadwick, Budd, Murchison, Simon, Acland, Buchanan, J.W. Russell and Benjamin Ward Richardson, put practical sanitation on a scientific basis. Even before the full demonstration of the germ theory, they had grasped the conception that the battle had to be fought against a living contagion which found in poverty, filth and wretched homes the conditions for its existence. One terrible disease was practically wiped out in twenty-five years of hard work. It is difficult to realize that within the memory of men now living, typhus fever was one of the great scourges of our large cities, and broke out in terrible epidemics—the most fatal of all to the medical profession. In the severe epidemic in Ireland in the forties of the last century, one fifth of all the doctors in the island died of typhus. A better idea of the new crusade, made possible by new knowledge, is to be had from a consideration of certain diseases against which the fight is in active progress.

Nothing illustrates more clearly the interdependence of the sciences than the reciprocal impulse given to new researches in pathology and entomology by the discovery of the part played by insects in the transmission of disease. The flea, the louse, the bedbug, the house fly, the mosquito, the tick, have all within a few years taken their places as important transmitters of disease. The fly population may be taken as the sanitary index of a place. The discovery, too, that insects are porters of disease has led to a great extension of our knowledge of their life history. Early in the nineties, when Dr. Thayer and I were busy with the study of malaria in Baltimore, we began experiments on the possible transmission of the parasites, and a tramp, who had been a medical student, offered himself as a subject. Before we began, Dr. Thayer sought information as to the varieties of mosquitoes known in America, but sought in vain: there had at that time been no systematic study. The fundamental study which set us on the track was a demonstration by Patrick Manson,(3) in 1879, of the association of filarian disease with the mosquito. Many observations had already been made, and were made subsequently, on the importance of insects as intermediary hosts in the animal parasites, but the first really great scientific demonstration of a widespread infection through insects was by Theobald Smith, now of Harvard University, in 1889, in a study of Texas fever of cattle.(4) I well remember the deep impression made upon me by his original communication, which in completeness, in accuracy of detail, in Harveian precision and in practical results remains one of the most brilliant pieces of experimental work ever undertaken. It is difficult to draw comparisons in pathology; but I think, if a census were taken among the world's workers on disease, the judgment to be based on the damage to health and direct mortality, the votes would be given to malaria as the greatest single destroyer of the human race. Cholera kills its thousands, plague, in its bad years, its hundreds of thousands, yellow fever, hookworm disease, pneumonia, tuberculosis, are all terribly destructive, some only in the tropics, others in more temperate regions: but malaria is today, as it ever was, a disease to which the word pandemic is specially applicable. In this country and in Europe, its ravages have lessened enormously during the past century, but in the tropics it is everywhere and always present, the greatest single foe of the white man, and at times and places it assumes the proportions of a terrible epidemic. In one district of India alone, during the last four months of 1908, one quarter of the total population suffered from the disease and there were 400,000 deaths—practically all from malaria. Today, the control of this terrible scourge is in our hands, and, as I shall tell you in a few minutes, largely because of this control, the Panama Canal is being built. No disease illustrates better the progressive evolution of scientific medicine. It is one of the oldest of known diseases. The Greeks and Graeco-Romans knew it well. It seems highly probable, as brought out by the studies of W.H.S. Jones of Cambridge, that, in part at least, the physical degeneration in Greece and Rome may have been due to the great increase of this disease. Its clinical manifestations were well known and admirably described by the older writers. In the seventeenth century, as I have already told you, the remarkable discovery was made that the bark of the cinchona tree was a specific. Between the date of the Countess's recovery in Lima and the year 1880 a colossal literature on the disease had accumulated. Literally thousands of workers had studied the various aspects of its many problems; the literature of this country, particularly of the Southern States, in the first half of the last century may be said to be predominantly malarial. Ordinary observation carried on for long centuries had done as much as was possible. In 1880, a young French army surgeon, Laveran by name, working in Algiers, found in the microscopic examination of the blood that there were little bodies in the red blood corpuscles, amoeboid in character, which he believed to be the germs of the disease. Very little attention at first was paid to his work, and it is not surprising. It was the old story of "Wolf, wolf"; there had been so many supposed "germs" that the profession had become suspicious. Several years elapsed before Surgeon-General Sternberg called the attention of the English-speaking world to Laveran's work: it was taken up actively in Italy, and in America by Councilman, Abbott and by others among us in Baltimore. The result of these widespread observations was the confirmation in every respect of Laveran's discovery of the association with malaria of a protozoan parasite. This was step number three. Clinical observation, empirical discovery of the cure, determination of the presence of a parasite. Two other steps followed rapidly. Another army surgeon, Ronald Ross, working in India, influenced by the work of Manson, proved that the disease was transmitted by certain varieties of mosquitoes. Experiments came in to support the studies in etiology; two of those may be quoted. Mosquitoes which had bitten malarial patients in Italy were sent to London and there allowed to bite Mr. Manson, son of Dr. Manson. This gentleman had not lived out of England, where there is now no acute malaria. He had been a perfectly healthy, strong man. In a few days following the bites of the infected mosquitoes, he had a typical attack of malarial fever.

(3) Journal Linnaean Society, London, 1879, XIV, 304-311.

(4) Medical News, Philadelphia, 1889, LV, 689-693, and monograph with Kilborne, Washington, 1893.

The other experiment, though of a different character, is quite as convincing. In certain regions about Rome, in the Campania, malaria is so prevalent that, in the autumn, almost everyone in the district is attacked, particularly if he is a newcomer. Dr. Sambon and a friend lived in this district from June 1 to September 1, 1900. The test was whether they could live in this exceedingly dangerous climate for the three months without catching malaria, if they used stringent precautions against the bites of mosquitoes. For this purpose the hut in which they lived was thoroughly wired, and they slept under netting. Both of these gentlemen, at the end of the period, had escaped the disease.

Then came the fifth and final triumph—the prevention of the disease. The anti-malarial crusade which has been preached by Sir Ronald Ross and has been carried out successfully on a wholesale scale in Italy and in parts of India and Africa, has reduced enormously the incidence of the disease. Professor Celli of Rome, in his lecture room, has an interesting chart which shows the reduction in the mortality from malaria in Italy since the preventive measures have been adopted—the deaths have fallen from above 28,000 in 1888 to below 2000 in 1910. There is needed a stirring campaign against the disease throughout the Southern States of this country.

The story of yellow fever illustrates one of the greatest practical triumphs of scientific medicine; indeed, in view of its far-reaching commercial consequences, it may range as one of the first achievements of the race. Ever since the discovery of America, the disease has been one of its great scourges, permanently endemic in the Spanish Main, often extending to the Southern States, occasionally into the North, and not infrequently it has crossed the Atlantic. The records of the British Army in the West Indies show an appalling death rate, chiefly from this disease. At Jamaica, for the twenty years ending in 1836, the average mortality was 101 per thousand, and in certain instances as high as 178. One of the most dreaded of all infections, the periods of epidemics in the Southern States have been the occasions of a widespread panic with complete paralysis of commerce. How appalling the mortality is may be judged from the outbreak in Philadelphia in 1793, when ten thousand people died in three months.(5) The epidemics in Spain in the early part of the nineteenth century were of great severity. A glance through La Roche's great book(6) on the subject soon gives one an idea of the enormous importance of the disease in the history of the Southern States. Havana, ever since its foundation, had been a hotbed of yellow fever. The best minds of the profession had been attracted to a solution of the problem, but all in vain. Commission after commission had been appointed, with negative results; various organisms had been described as the cause, and there were sad illustrations of the tragedy associated with investigations undertaken without proper training or proper technique. By the year 1900, not only had the ground been cleared, but the work on insect-borne disease by Manson and by Ross had given observers an important clue. It had repeatedly been suggested that some relation existed between the bites of mosquitoes and the tropical fevers, particularly by that remarkable student, Nott of Mobile, and the French physician, Beauperthuy. But the first to announce clearly the mosquito theory of the disease was Carlos Finlay of Havana. Early in the spring of 1900, during the occupation of Cuba by the United States, a commission appointed by Surgeon-General Sternberg (himself one of the most energetic students of the disease) undertook fresh investigations. Dr. Walter Reed, Professor of Bacteriology in the Army Medical School, was placed in charge: Dr. Carroll of the United States Army, Dr. Agramonte of Havana and Dr. Jesse W. Lazear were the other members. At the Johns Hopkins Hospital, we were deeply interested in the work, as Dr. Walter Reed was a favorite pupil of Professor Welch, a warm friend of all of us, and a frequent visitor to our laboratories. Dr. Jesse Lazear, who had been my house physician, had worked with Dr. Thayer and myself at malaria, and gave up the charge of my clinical laboratory to join the commission.

(5) Matthew Carey: A Short Account of the Malignant Fever, Philadelphia, 1793.

(6) R. La Roche: Yellow Fever, 2 vols., Philadelphia, 1855.

Many scientific discoveries have afforded brilliant illustrations of method in research, but in the work of these men one is at a loss to know which to admire more—the remarkable accuracy and precision of the experiments, or the heroism of the men—officers and rank and file of the United States Army; they knew all the time that they were playing with death, and some of them had to pay the penalty! The demonstration was successful—beyond peradventure—that yellow fever could be transmitted by mosquitoes, and equally the negative proposition—that it could not be transmitted by fomites. An interval of twelve or more days was found to be necessary after the mosquito has bitten a yellow fever patient before it is capable of transmitting the infection. Lazear permitted himself to be bitten by a stray mosquito while conducting his experiments in the yellow fever hospital. Bitten on the thirteenth, he sickened on the eighteenth and died on the twenty-fifth of September, but not until he had succeeded in showing in two instances that mosquitoes could convey the infection. He added another to the long list of members of the profession who have laid down their lives in search of the causes of disease. Of such men as Lazear and of Myers of the Liverpool Yellow-Fever Commission, Dutton and young Manson, may fitly be sung from the noblest of American poems the tribute which Lowell paid to Harvard's sons who fell in the War of Secession:

Many in sad faith sought for her,
Many with crossed hands sighed for her;
But these, our brothers, fought for her,
At life's dear peril wrought for her,
So loved her that they died for her.

Fortunately, the commander-in-chief at the time in Cuba was General Leonard Wood, who had been an army surgeon, and he was the first to appreciate the importance of the discovery. The sanitation of Havana was placed in the hands of Dr. Gorgas, and within nine months the city was cleared of yellow fever, and, with the exception of a slight outbreak after the withdrawal of the American troops, has since remained free from a disease which had been its scourge for centuries. As General Wood remarked, "Reed's discovery has resulted in the saving of more lives annually than were lost in the Cuban War, and saves the commercial interest of the world a greater financial loss each year than the cost of the Cuban War. He came to Cuba at a time when one third of the officers of my staff died of yellow fever, and we were discouraged at the failure of our efforts to control it." Following the example of Havana other centres were attacked, at Vera Cruz and in Brazil, with the same success, and it is safe to say that now, thanks to the researches of Reed and his colleagues, with proper measures, no country need fear a paralyzing outbreak of this once dreaded disease.

The scientific researches in the last two decades of the nineteenth century made possible the completion of the Panama Canal. The narrow isthmus separating the two great oceans and joining the two great continents, has borne for four centuries an evil repute as the White Man's Grave. Silent upon a peak of Darien, stout Cortez with eagle eye had gazed on the Pacific. As early as 1520, Saavedra proposed to cut a canal through the Isthmus. There the first city was founded by the conquerors of the new world, which still bears the name of Panama. Spaniards, English and French fought along its coasts; to it the founder of the Bank of England took his ill-fated colony; Raleigh, Drake, Morgan the buccaneer, and scores of adventurers seeking gold, found in fever an enemy stronger than the Spaniard. For years the plague-stricken Isthmus was abandoned to the negroes and the half-breeds, until in 1849, stimulated by the gold fever of California, a railway was begun by the American engineers, Totten and Trautwine, and completed in 1855, a railway every tie of which cost the life of a man. The dream of navigators and practical engineers was taken in hand by Ferdinand de Lesseps in January, 1881. The story of the French Canal Company is a tragedy unparalleled in the history of finance, and, one may add, in the ravages of tropical disease. Yellow fever, malaria, dysentery, typhus, carried off in nine years nearly twenty thousand employees. The mortality frequently rose above 100, sometimes to 130, 140 and in September, 1885, it reached the appalling figure of 176.97 per thousand work people. This was about the maximum death rate of the British Army in the West Indies in the nineteenth century.

When, in 1904, the United States undertook to complete the Canal, everyone felt that the success or failure was largely a matter of sanitary control. The necessary knowledge existed, but under the circumstances could it be made effective? Many were doubtful. Fortunately, there was at the time in the United States Army a man who had already served an apprenticeship in Cuba, and to whom more than to anyone else was due the disappearance of yellow fever from that island. To a man, the profession in the United States felt that could Dr. Gorgas be given full control of the sanitary affairs of the Panama Zone, the health problem, which meant the Canal problem, could be solved. There was at first a serious difficulty relating to the necessary administrative control by a sanitary officer. In an interview which Dr. Welch and I had with President Roosevelt, he keenly felt this difficulty and promised to do his best to have it rectified. It is an open secret that at first, as was perhaps only natural, matters did not go very smoothly, and it took a year or more to get properly organized. Yellow fever recurred on the Isthmus in 1904 and in the early part of 1905. It was really a colossal task in itself to undertake the cleaning of the city of Panama, which had been for centuries a pesthouse, the mortality in which, even after the American occupation, reached during one month the rate of 71 per thousand living. There have been a great many brilliant illustrations of the practical application of science in preserving the health of a community and in saving life, but it is safe to say that, considering the circumstances, the past history, and the extraordinary difficulties to be overcome, the work accomplished by the Isthmian Canal Commission is unique. The year 1905 was devoted to organization; yellow fever was got rid of, and at the end of the year the total mortality among the whites had fallen to 8 per thousand, but among the blacks it was still high, 44. For three years, with a progressively increasing staff which had risen to above 40,000, of whom more than 12,000 were white, the death rate progressively fell.

Of the six important tropical diseases, plague, which reached the Isthmus one year, was quickly held in check. Yellow fever, the most dreaded of them all, never recurred. Beri-beri, which in 1906 caused sixty-eight deaths, has gradually disappeared. The hookworm disease, ankylostomiasis, has steadily decreased. From the very outset, malaria has been taken as the measure of sanitary efficiency. Throughout the French occupation it was the chief enemy to be considered, not only because of its fatality, but on account of the prolonged incapacity following infection. In 1906, out of every 1000 employees there were admitted to the hospital from malaria 821; in 1907, 424; in 1908, 282; in 1912, 110; in 1915, 51; in 1917, 14. The fatalities from the disease have fallen from 233 in 1906 to 154 in 1907, to 73 in 1908 and to 7 in 1914. The death rate for malarial fever per 1000 population sank from 8.49 in 1906 to 0.11 in 1918. Dysentery, next to malaria the most serious of the tropical diseases in the Zone, caused 69 deaths in 1906; 48 in 1907; in 1908, with nearly 44,000, only 16 deaths, and in 1914, 4.(*) But it is when the general figures are taken that we see the extraordinary reduction that has taken place. Out of every 1000 engaged in 1908 only a third of the number died that died in 1906, and half the number that died in 1907.

(*) Figures for recent years supplied by editors.

In 1914, the death rate from disease among white males had fallen to 3.13 per thousand. The rate among the 2674 American women and children connected with the Commission was only 9.72 per thousand. But by far the most gratifying reduction is among the blacks, among whom the rate from disease had fallen to the surprisingly low figure in 1912 of 8.77 per thousand; in 1906 it was 47 per thousand. A remarkable result is that in 1908 the combined tropical diseases—malaria, dysentery and beri-beri—killed fewer than the two great killing diseases of the temperate zone, pneumonia and tuberculosis—127 in one group and 137 in the other. The whole story is expressed in two words, EFFECTIVE ORGANIZA-TICN, and the special value of this experiment in sanitation is that it has been made, and made successfully, in one of the great plague spots of the world.

Month by month a little, gray-covered pamphlet was published by Colonel Gorgas, a "Report of the Department of Sanitation of the Isthmian Canal Commission." I have been one of the favored to whom it has been sent year by year, and, keenly interested as I have always been in infectious diseases, and particularly in malaria and dysentery, I doubt if anyone has read it more faithfully. In evidence of the extraordinary advance made in sanitation by Gorgas, I give a random example from one of his monthly reports (1912): In a population of more than 52,000, the death rate from disease had fallen to 7.31 per thousand; among the whites it was 2.80 and among the colored people 8.77. Not only is the profession indebted to Colonel Gorgas and his staff for this remarkable demonstration, but they have offered an example of thoroughness and efficiency which has won the admiration of the whole world. As J. E. Bishop, secretary of the Isthmian Canal Commission, has recently said: "The Americans arrived on the Isthmus in the full light of these two invaluable discoveries (the insect transmission of yellow fever and malaria). Scarcely had they begun active work when an outbreak of yellow fever occurred which caused such a panic throughout their force that nothing except the lack of steamship accommodation prevented the flight of the entire body from the Isthmus. Prompt, intelligent and vigorous application of the remedies shown to be effective by the mosquito discoveries not only checked the progress of the pest, but banished it forever from the Isthmus. In this way, and in this alone, was the building of the canal made possible. The supreme credit for its construction therefore belongs to the brave men, surgeons of the United States Army, who by their high devotion to duty and to humanity risked their lives in Havana in 1900-1901 to demonstrate the truth of the mosquito theory. "(7)

(7) Bishop: The French at Panama, Scribner's Magazine, January, 1913, p. 42.

One disease has still a special claim upon the public in this country. Some fourteen or fifteen years ago, in an address on the problem of typhoid fever in the United States, I contended that the question was no longer in the hands of the profession. In season and out of season we had preached salvation from it in volumes which fill state reports, public health journals and the medical periodicals. Though much has been done, typhoid fever remains a question of grave national concern. You lost in this state(7a) in 1911 from typhoid fever 154 lives, every one sacrificed needlessly, every one a victim of neglect and incapacity. Between 1200 and 1500 persons had a slow, lingering illness. A nation of contradictions and paradoxes—a clean people, by whom personal hygiene is carefully cultivated, but it has displayed in matters of public sanitation a carelessness simply criminal: a sensible people, among whom education is more widely diffused than in any other country, supinely acquiesces in conditions often shameful beyond expression. The solution of the problem is not very difficult. What has been done elsewhere can be done here. It is not so much in the cities, though here too the death rate is still high, but in the smaller towns and rural districts, in many of which the sanitary conditions are still those of the Middle Ages. How Galen would have turned up his nose with contempt at the water supply of the capital of the Dominion of Canada, scourged so disgracefully by typhoid fever of late! There is no question that the public is awakening, but many State Boards of Health need more efficient organization, and larger appropriations. Others are models, and it is not for lack of example that many lag behind. The health officers should have special training in sanitary science and special courses leading to diplomas in public health should be given in the medical schools. Were the health of the people made a question of public and not of party policy, only a skilled expert could possibly be appointed as a public health officer, not, as is now so often the case, the man with the political pull.

(7a) Connecticut.

It is a long and tragic story in the annals of this country. That distinguished man, the first professor of physic in this University in the early years of last century, Dr. Nathan Smith, in that notable monograph on "Typhus Fever" (1824), tells how the disease had followed him in his various migrations, from 1787, when he began to practice, all through his career, and could he return this year, in some hundred and forty or one hundred and fifty families of the state he would find the same miserable tragedy which he had witnessed so often in the same heedless sacrifice of the young on the altar of ignorance and incapacity.

TUBERCULOSIS

IN a population of about one million, seventeen hundred persons died of tuberculosis in this state in the year 1911—a reduction in thirty years of nearly 50 per cent. A generation has changed completely our outlook on one of the most terrible scourges of the race. It is simply appalling to think of the ravages of this disease in civilized communities. Before the discovery by Robert Koch of the bacillus, we were helpless and hopeless; in an Oriental fatalism we accepted with folded hands a state of affairs which use and wont had made bearable. Today, look at the contrast! We are both helpful and hopeful. Knowing the cause of the disease, knowing how it is distributed, better able to recognize the early symptoms, better able to cure a very considerable portion of all early cases, we have gradually organized an enthusiastic campaign which is certain to lead to victory. The figures I have quoted indicate how progressively the mortality is falling. Only, do not let us be disappointed if this comparatively rapid fall is not steadily maintained in the country at large. It is a long fight against a strong enemy, and at the lowest estimate it will take several generations before tuberculosis is placed at last, with leprosy and typhus, among the vanquished diseases. Education, organization, cooperation—these are the weapons of our warfare. Into details I need not enter. The work done by the National Association under the strong guidance of its secretary, Mr. Farrand, the pioneer studies of Trudeau and the optimism which he has brought into the campaign, the splendid demonstration by the New York Board of Health of what organization can do, have helped immensely in this worldwide conflict.

SOME years ago, in an address at Edinburgh, I spoke of the triple gospel which man has published—of his soul, of his goods, of his body. This third gospel, the gospel of his body, which brings man into relation with nature, has been a true evangelion, the glad tidings of the final conquest of nature by which man has redeemed thousands of his fellow men from sickness and from death.

If, in the memorable phrase of the Greek philosopher, Prodicus, "That which benefits human life is God," we may see in this new gospel a link betwixt us and the crowning race of those who eye to eye shall look on knowledge, and in whose hand nature shall be an open book—an approach to the glorious day of which Shelley sings so gloriously:

Happiness
And Science dawn though late upon the earth;
Peace cheers the mind, health renovates the frame;
Disease and pleasure cease to mingle here,
Reason and passion cease to combat there,
Whilst mind unfettered o'er the earth extends
Its all-subduing energies, and wields
The sceptre of a vast dominion there.

(Daemon of the World, Pt. II.)